Just having lost my husband to a massive MI, I was unable after a couple chapters. I had to skip to the chapter on risks. I did this and was profoundly struck by how exact my husband's risks, heredity and lifestyle choices were mirrored. It was almost as if he was the model for that chapter. I was emotionally impacted by how much Jim knew about his risk factors and regretfully, how much he might not have known and would have gained from your book. I know neither of us knew as much as I read in that one chapter. I then went to the chapter on women's heart and read very carefully. I also have risks and family history but I have the chance to stay healthy and change what I need to change. I feel more informed. Despite being an RN, I only focused on my current personal situation. I had to digest some of the info and emotions I felt — a step at a time. Thank you. Ann Noland, RN, President and CEO May Creek Senior Living Campus

Heart disease is the leading cause of death in the United States. Dr. Kuffel's book gives the layperson a guide to understanding how coronary artery disease develops and offers ways to help avoid it through lifestyle changes. The sections on nutrition are cutting edge and have the potential to prevent and sometimes even reverse coronary disease. I commend Dr. Kuffel for providing vital facts about prevention, which are often neglected. To become familiar with ways to prevent disease is a great gift that leads to a longer, healthier life. Barbara Palmer, Screenwriter, Plant-based health advocate

Your Heart is a wonderful guide for any individual wishing to achieve cardiac health. In this book, Dr. Kuffel describes the emotion and history of heartfelt care in combination with current scientific and clinical information. Through her clear and concise style she makes this very important subject both accessible and understandable to the lay and professional person alike. Read it for your heart's sake! Maura Fields, RN, Chief Clinical Officer, North Valley Hospital

Your Heart is the book I wish had been available five years ago when my husband "flat-lined" during a catastrophic heart attack. Emergency surgery saved him, but our lives changed forever. Panicked and overwhelmed by a million questions I didn't know how to ask, I would have welcomed Dr. Kuffel's clear explanations of what went wrong, what the surgeon did to fix it, and how to make major diet changes. The book is easy to read. Even when the author offers scientific documentation, she wisely recognizes many readers may not want to plow through complicated chemistry, and reassures them that it's okay to "skip ahead to the next section." She also reviews the latest studies which have changed some conventional wisdoms in treatment and prevention. This is the first book I grab any time a question comes up regarding heart health. — An invaluable resource and practical guide for anyone who has a heart. Deb Burke Author, editor, wife of survivor

Your book is chocked full of information everyone should know. This is an excellent one-source reference on the human heart complete with descriptions of the heart's function, ailments and current treatments. Perhaps most importantly, it details preventative measures to maintain a healthy heart. — I recommend this book as a guide to anyone interested in living a longer, healthier life. Thank you for writing *Your Heart.* Brenda Erickson, MN Department of Human Services Supervisor

Your Heart provides concise information about how the heart functions, prevention of heart disease, and critical signs of heart problems. I was particularly interested in Dr. Kuffel's description of heart disease in women and surprised to learn that symptoms of a heart attack can differ dramatically from what men experience. As a woman with heart disease on both sides of the family, I feel better prepared to manage my heart health after reading *Your Heart.* Ann Minnett, Author *Burden of Breath*

This compact guidebook expands knowledge of specific heart-problem diagnoses and interventions that would have been a valuable resource during my husband's four heart procedures. A broadened understanding inspired us to change from harmful to good habits that can actually reverse heart disease. Barb

Greenside, Past Human Resources Administrator – University. of Northwestern - St. Paul

This great up-to-date guidebook is a perfect way to learn the importance of understanding risks for heart disease and how to make changes in your life to live healthier. Weaving in stories of real people and how they met with the shock of heart attacks and undiagnosed health problems makes this important book not only a solid health reference, it is readable and personal. Lavonne Mueller, playwright, author of *Hotel Splendid*

YOUR HEART:
Prevent and Reverse Heart Disease in Women, Men and Children

Betty Kuffel, MD, FACP

YourHeartBook.com

Cover and Drawings by Blue Heron Loft

Publisher: Lipstick Logic LLP™

Published in the United States of America

ISBN-13: 978-1490483603

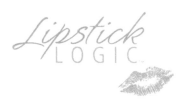

Founded by two sisters, Lipstick Logic LLP was developed to bring health education to women. Because some of the most serious health problems, including heart disease and obesity also affect men and children, the first two Lipstick Logic books are written for everyone: women, men and children.

To explain the meaning behind the lip print, we'd like to share our Lipstick Logic motto:

"Symbolic of the individuality of each woman's life, this lip print represents each woman's unique story. By changing lip colors, a woman can change her appearance. By making new choices, she can change her life."

Our goal is to provide current science-based information to provide a sound foundation for health decisions.

CONTENTS
PART ONE
CARDIOVASCULAR DISEASE:
THE HEART AND ARTERIES

i

Your Heart

Betty Kuffel, MD

Your Heart

"This is 9-1-1. What is your emergency?"
"It's my wife. Help me. She's not breathing!"

An ambulance radio call to the emergency room staff broke the early morning silence. "Regional ER, this is Medic One."

A voice answered, "Regional ER here. — Go ahead, Medic One."

"Medic-One is inbound to your facility Code 3. Break." — The breathless voice continued, "CPR in progress, 51 year-old female. Witnessed arrest after awakening with chest pain. CPR started by husband. Unsuccessful shocks en route."

Moments later, a distant siren drew closer and abruptly stopped as the Medic One vehicle arrived at the ambulance entrance. Doors parted. The waiting ER Code Team helped medics roll the patient into a large treatment room while continuing oxygen and chest compressions.

The paramedic reported, "Dr. Kuffel, this is Dorothy Jackson. She's had three rounds of drugs, three shocks. V-fib and V-tach — got a rhythm back, but we lost it."

Across America, calls similar to this are received in emergency centers every day. Unfortunately, the first symptom of heart disease is often sudden death. Half of all deaths from heart attacks occur outside the hospital. Many men and women do not even know they have heart disease, yet die suddenly from cardiac arrest — their hearts simply stop.

How can anyone have advanced heart disease and not know it? — At first, there are no symptoms. In fact there may be no symptoms with an artery that is 90% blocked! Slow but progressive narrowing of the *coronary arteries* that supply the heart muscle with oxygen occurs over many years and is the leading cause of death in both men and women.

When symptoms begin, they may seem insignificant and unrelated to the heart. We usually think of chest pain as a warning sign of heart disease or a heart attack, often it is. Among both men and women, the classic symptoms of an impending heart attack are:

- Chest discomfort (sometimes with pain or pressure extending into the neck, jaw or arms)

1

- Upper abdominal discomfort and nausea, "indigestion"
- Perspiration and shortness of breath
- Upper back pain

Dorothy's personal history is common. About twenty pounds overweight and taking no medications, she was a non-smoker, yet she suffered a cardiac arrest. Her husband said, "She has never been sick a day in her life. Dorothy hasn't visited a doctor since the birth of our son 15 years ago."

Fortunately, Dorothy's husband called 9-1-1 and immediately began performing chest compressions. He had taken a CPR course and knew what to do. C-P-R stands for Cardio-Pulmonary-Resuscitation. Anyone can perform this life-saving procedure. Additional CPR information is provided at the end of Chapter 7.

In the ER environment, when a "Code" is called, it usually means a patient is in crisis and more help is needed. Often, someone has stopped breathing or has had a cardiac arrest. The Code Team rushes to take their positions, ready to provide assistance. Most teams include doctors, nurses, respiratory therapists, laboratory technicians, pharmacists and X-ray techs. With a flurry of activity, they begin performing their pre-designated responsibilities. In Dorothy's case, a heart specialist and the heart cath-lab team were also alerted.

Dorothy survived. After a tube in her airway provided more oxygen to her lungs, shocks reorganized her heart rhythm; medications raised her blood pressure and calmed her irritable heart. She received blood thinners and a trip to the heart cath-lab. There, the heart specialist inserted a tiny catheter to dilate the closed artery in her heart and placed a stent to prop it open. Because Dorothy's brain suffered injury due to inadequate circulation and lack of oxygen when her heart stopped, she remained unresponsive. Her heart function normalized but it wasn't clear if she would recover.

In the intensive care unit, connected to a ventilator helping her breathe, doctors cooled her body to protect her brain from swelling. Later, and after gradual re-warming, her brain function improved. Two weeks later, Dorothy went home with medications, heart health information and an exercise and rehabilitation plan.

Your Heart

Even when coronary disease has narrowed arteries and obstructed blood flow to the heart, treatment is possible. There is hope. There is even hope for reversing the disease.

Cardiovascular Disease

Coronary arteries carry blood, nutrients and oxygen to the heart muscle. When waxy cholesterol accumulates within the inner artery wall, it stiffens the artery and begins blocking the flow of blood. The artery disease is called *atherosclerosis.* The word describes what is happening: *athero* means fat; *sclerosis* means hardening. Many people call atherosclerosis "hardening of the arteries."

Because this destructive process occurs not only in the heart arteries, but in arteries throughout the body, it is called *cardiovascular disease.* When blood flow is decreased to other organs, such as the kidneys and brain, kidney failure and dementia occur.

Many other forms of heart disease are the result of infection, toxins, hereditary factors and congenital abnormalities over which you have little control. But with the right information, you can take control and treat atherosclerosis. The sooner you make good decisions to improve your health, the more likely you are to add years to your life. Food choices play a huge role. Both men and women are developing coronary artery disease at younger ages. Early evidence of coronary artery disease is even seen in children.

Beginning at a young age, what you eat makes a huge difference. Arteries are more likely to become narrowed throughout the entire body if predominant food choices are:
- High in salt, fat and calories — such as potato chips and French fries.
- High in sugar — such as sweet-rolls, pancakes and candy.
- High in saturated fats — such as bacon cheese-burgers.

Many factors contribute to coronary artery disease; smoking and *uncontrolled* high blood pressure are two of the most harmful. In the US each year, these two factors are responsible for one-in-five heart related deaths. Next are obesity and inactivity, accounting for approximately one-in-ten heart deaths per year.

Experts agree inflammation is the likely trigger for atherosclerosis. Diabetes, obesity and inactivity are directly related to developing atherosclerosis. Other factors include: high LDL-cholesterol, stress, excessive alcohol intake, and illicit drug use. All of them increase inflammation in the body. Blood tests can measure inflammatory markers that correlate with coronary artery disease.

Daily stress levels rise with holding a job while juggling household responsibilities and securing childcare. Job burn-out, job loss, depression, sleeplessness and anxiety, all raise blood pressure and add to heart disease risks. Additionally, working the night shift adds to serious health problems including heart disease, diabetes and obesity.

Gender makes a difference. Men tend to develop coronary artery disease years earlier than women. Younger, premenopausal estrogen-producing women are typically at lower coronary disease risk than men the same age because estrogen is protective. As postmenopausal women age, *their risks soon equal those in men.*

This guide will take you through body processes contributing to the coronary artery disease epidemic and provide accurate science-based information about actions to improve your health. Even if you already have been diagnosed with coronary artery disease, you have the ability to stop its progression. Aggressive treatment can reverse changes inside the artery wall.

Remember — prevention is always the best medicine.

Your Heart

Chapter 1
Heart Anatomy and Function

Heart Structure and Circulation

By understanding normal function of the cardiovascular system, you will better understand what happens when something goes wrong. Even though the human heart is not shaped like a valentine, it is central to descriptions of caring, commitment and in thoughts of love. This biological engine is about the size of a clenched fist. It is composed of four compartments and a complex tangle of tubes. Angled leftward, the heart sits in the center of the chest between the lungs.

About seventy times a minute, spontaneous pacemaker cells fire off an electrical impulse signaling the muscle to contract. The contraction squeezes blood into the lungs and out the aorta to the rest of the body, generating the "heart beat." The heart is the only muscle that never rests.

The heart has four chambers, two upper and two lower:
- The upper chambers are the right atrium and the left atrium. They are separated by a wall called the atrial septum.
- The lower and larger chambers are the right and the left ventricles. They are separated by a wall called the ventricular septum. Each ventricle has two one-way doors called heart valves.
- The interior areas of the ventricles are the same size, but the left ventricle muscle is stronger to provide the necessary strength to pump blood out to the body.
- The atrial septum and the ventricular septum separate de-oxygenated blood on the right from oxygenated blood on the left.

Four valves direct the flow of blood in one direction:
- Blood flows from the right atrium through the *tricuspid valve* into the right ventricle.

5

- The right ventricle pumps blood through the *pulmonary valve* into the pulmonary artery and into the lungs.
- Blood flows from the lungs to the left atrium, then to the left ventricle through the *mitral valve*.
- The left ventricle pumps blood through the *aortic valve* into the aorta and out to the body.

Blood circulates via two primary types of vessels called arteries and veins. They are interconnected at the tissue level by a vast collection of tiny capillaries. Vessels near the heart are large. They become smaller and smaller the farther they extend away from the heart.

Arteries carry oxygen-rich blood from the lungs to the rest of the body. Structurally, arteries have muscular walls that expand and relax with each beat of the heart. As blood is pushed out of the heart, these pliable walls bulge with each beat and create your pulse. A heart rate too slow, too fast or irregular indicates a heart problem.

♥ **What to do: Learn to count your pulse.**

To count your pulse: turn your right palm up. Press the second and third fingers of your left hand on your right wrist along the thumb side. Find the pulsation and count each beat for a full minute. That is your heart rate per minute; around 70 beats per minute is a normal rate.

Capillaries form the interconnection between *arterioles* (tiny arteries) and *venules* (tiny veins). In the expansive network of capillaries, nutrients and oxygen are supplied to tissues and waste products are removed.

Veins are thin non-pulsating blood vessels with delicate one-way valves spaced along their interior surface. Veins carry de-oxygenated blood away from the capillaries back to the heart through larger and larger veins until reaching either of the two largest veins, the inferior or the superior vena cava that connect to the right atrium. From there, blood enters the lungs and travels through lung capillaries to obtain a new supply of oxygen and expel the carbon dioxide.

Primary blood components are:
- Plasma – a yellowish fluid that makes up 55% of the blood volume. It carries many blood cells including

platelets, white and red cells, along with: glucose, proteins, electrolytes, clotting factors, hormones, blood-fats bound to protein carriers and metabolic waste products.

- Red blood cells – the oxygen-carrying cells that make up 45% of blood volume.
- White blood cells – many types of infection-fighting cells that together make up about 1% of the blood.
- Platelets – tiny powerful blood cells that initiate blood clotting.

Bodily functions are intricately meshed. Even a few days without water results in tissue damage, kidney failure and death. Along with transporting red blood cells that carry oxygen to all organs, the red superhighway carries fluids filled with nutrients to feed all cells. Swirling throughout the body are cells that support life functions, fight infection, and promote clotting. The blood also carries factors that, in excess, cause heart disease and early death.

In discussing cardiovascular disease, we are primarily concerned with coronary arteries, but the lymphatic vessels are also transporters of essential life-sustaining elements. The cardiovascular and lymph systems interact to move fluids through the body. Thin-walled branching lymph vessels called lymphatics direct lymph fluid from each side of the body and flow into large veins near the heart.

Key organs in the lymph system where immune responses are regulated are: the thymus, spleen and lymph nodes. Because lymph fluid drains areas where the body mounts attacks against invading bacteria or viruses, this fluid also carries antibodies, organisms and toxic byproducts. Lymph fluid percolates through the liver. From the digestive tract, lymph fluid transports nutrients, fats and fat-soluble vitamins into the blood for circulation and distribution.

The Blood's Superhighway
Next, a journey along the superhighway will help explain the blood-circuit through the heart, to the body and back to the heart again. You will also learn how the intricate coronary arteries provide blood to the heart muscle. Take a few minutes to study the heart diagram below. It shows heart chambers,

valves and the direction of flow as blood leaves and returns to the heart.

When looking at X-rays or medical drawings, the right side of the image/person is on the left side of the picture; the left side of the person/image is on the right side of the picture.

Imagine you are looking at a person facing you. In the drawing, the heart is cut through the center to show the chambers, valves and great vessels.

With each beat of the heart, blood is pushed along the superhighway into the lungs or out to the body. For simplicity, we will follow blood as it leaves the left side of the heart and returns to the right side of the heart.

Fasten your seatbelts for a trip through the heart. Here we go!

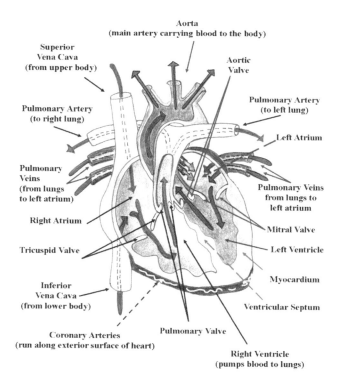

8

Your Heart

Newly oxygenated bright red blood leaves the lungs and travels through the pulmonary veins to the left atrium. From the left atrium, the blood flows into the left ventricle through a one-way door called the *mitral valve*. When the ventricle contracts, the mitral valve snaps shut to stop the blood from backwashing into the atrium. Blood in the left ventricle now spurts forward through the *aortic valve* into the aorta and out to the body. This large artery divides into branches allowing blood to surge to the upper body and brain, and down to the abdomen, intestines and lower body.

As the aorta extends away from the heart, it divides into the smaller branches much the way limbs of trees grow outward into twigs. The smallest arteries, the arterioles connect to the capillary network where tissues receive nutrients from the blood. At the far end, the capillaries become the smallest veins called venules.

All along this superhighway, cellular exchanges occur between the blood, the organs and tissues. The exchanges deplete the blood of oxygen and nutrients while collecting carbon dioxide and other waste products from cells.

Reaching the venule level, the deoxygenated "blue" blood begins its journey back to the heart as it travels through larger and larger veins, until arriving at the inferior and superior vena cavae. From there, blood empties into the right atrium en route to the lungs to take up more oxygen.

The right atrium receives the *blue blood* carrying waste products. The blood is referred to as blue because it appears darker in color after the red blood cells have been stripped of their oxygen by cells in muscle and other tissue along the superhighway route. From the right atrium, blood travels through the *tricuspid valve* into the right ventricle. There it is pumped through the *pulmonary valve* into a large pulmonary artery which divides and carries blood to each lung.

When valves are defective, they do not close and open properly, producing a whooshing sound heard with a stethoscope when listening to the chest over the heart. The abnormal sound called a *heart murmur* is from turbulent blood flow, much like that created when river water rushes over rocks. Diseased valves may allow blood to backwash. Sometimes, a diseased valve will act like a stuck door that doesn't fully open, partially blocking the forward flow of

9

blood. Murmurs may be mild and cause no functional problems. Others may require interventions or replacement.

Blood passing through lung capillaries receives oxygen and releases carbon dioxide. The red blood cells are aligned like boxcars to upload and transport oxygen to all cells in the body. The exchange of gases occurs when oxygen moves into the red cells from tiny air pockets containing the air you breathe called *alveoli*. Carbon dioxide moves into the alveoli and is exhaled.

Before oxygenated blood can be carried from the lung tissue throughout the body to where it is needed, the pulmonary veins must first carry it back to the left atrium.

You can now unfasten your seat belt, — you have traveled the blood circuit through the body. This entire process repeats itself over and over again, allowing oxygen-rich blood from the lungs to pour out of the left heart and travel through arteries to the rest of the body and return via veins to be re-oxygenated once again. The average circulation time for one red cell to make the round trip is 60 seconds, except for cells traveling through complex organs like the liver where it takes a few minutes.

Don't be concerned if you didn't follow every aspect of the blood's route. Simply stated, blood flows right to left, through the lungs to pick up oxygen for the next circuit. This life-sustaining process happens continuously throughout every minute of life.

The main circulation route is complete. Next, you will see how the heart muscle is nourished even as it works constantly to pump blood throughout the body.

Coronary Artery Circulation

Two main heart arteries originate from the aorta, just outside the aortic valve. Variations in coronary anatomy occur, but in most cases the left coronary artery supplies much of the front and left heart. The right coronary artery supplies the right side and circles around to the back of the heart. Both of these large surface arteries subdivide into smaller and smaller branches that penetrate and feed the heart wall.

When the heart relaxes between contractions, blood fills the ventricle preparing for the next beat. During this period, the relaxed muscle allows oxygen-rich blood from the coronary surface arteries to enter the smaller arteries and arterioles to feed the heart wall and reach the heart capillaries.

At the capillary level, oxygen and nutrients are supplied to the ever-working heart muscle. Most of the deoxygenated blood from heart capillaries is carried away from the heart to the right atrium via veins. These veins follow the coronary arteries along the surface of the heart and merge with the *coronary sinus*, a larger vein that flows into the right atrium. Some of the smallest veins drain directly into any of the four heart chambers.

What Makes Coronary Arteries So Important?

The heart needs continuous nourishment of oxygen-rich blood. When coronary arteries become diseased from the buildup of cholesterol plaques inside their walls, blood flow decreases. Without adequate circulation, *ischemia* causes chest discomfort, *angina*. Ischemia is the term used to describe restriction of blood supply and oxygen to tissues.

Due to poor lifestyle, unhealthy food choices, lack of exercise, and hereditary factors, this preventable disease of the coronary arteries develops over years. Smooth interior artery walls gradually become roughened with an accumulation of cholesterol lumps called *plaques*. The interior becomes smaller and smaller until blood is unable to pass. At times, a clot forms over a rough area completely blocking the narrowed vessel.

Sometimes, the rough surface of a cholesterol plaque inside the artery abruptly breaks open and releases pieces of cholesterol into the blood. Clot or cholesterol particles are carried along in the blood until they lodge and fully block a coronary artery. The blockage cuts off blood flow beyond, starving the heart muscle of oxygen. When a vessel is blocked, by plaque, a clot or cholesterol particles, a heart attack occurs.

Heart attacks are called "MIs" by many medical practitioners. *MI* is short for *myocardial infarction. Myo* pertains to muscle, *cardial* pertains to the heart, and *infarction* means tissue death due to lack of oxygen.

As in Dorothy's case, if a heart attack occurs, rapid interventions to open the artery and restore blood flow can be life-saving. If flow is not quickly restored in the area beyond the blockage, cells die.

When heart cells are damaged by the lack of oxygen and nutrients, the dying cells leak *troponin*. Rising troponin levels in the blood indicate a heart attack has occurred. Dying cells become irritable and abnormal rhythms develop. The heart muscle may weaken and begin to fail. Depending on location and size of the damaged area, risks for death and disability vary.

EXTERNAL HEART
Plaque Build-Up and Blood Clot in Coronary Artery

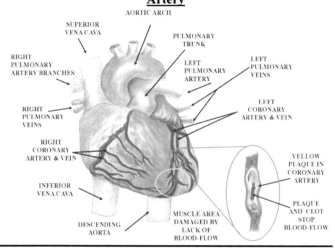

Your Heart

Changes at the Cellular Level

Early findings in coronary arteries are thickening and fatty streaks as atherosclerosis develops inside vessel walls. Within the fatty streaks, two primary white cell types accumulate: *macrophages* and *T-lymphocytes.* Macrophages are scavenger cells that typically remove cell wastes by ingesting and degrading them. When macrophages become engorged with fat particles they are called "foam cells" because of their appearance. An accelerated inflammatory response against the fat-filled cells occurs, promoting plaque development. A fibrous lattice formation develops and acts as a stabilizer to the plaque allowing even more cholesterol to accumulate.

Over years, plaques increase in size to the point of impeding blood flow. Arteries start out smooth and elastic. Through destructive changes, they stiffen and may even become calcified. Both T-lymphocytes and macrophages are seen in all stages of arterial plaque development. Their presence is indicative of an active inflammatory process.

The complex atherosclerosis process is magnified in inflammatory conditions such as diabetes. It is also increased in people diagnosed with lupus, psoriasis and other autoimmune diseases when the body produces antibodies against itself. Cell biologists continue to examine the relationships between the macrophages, T-lymphocytes, LDL cholesterol and other molecular components of cholesterol plaques. The hope would be to identify the exact trigger and disable the process before damage occurs.

Cholesterol comes in many forms; they are all lipids. *Lipid* is the medical term for "fat" within the blood stream. A lipid blood panel measures many different cholesterol molecules. LDL cholesterol is a destructive form found in artery plaques. A blood test measuring the inflammatory marker C–Reactive Protein may also be done to help evaluate the risks of disease development.

Statin drugs attack the core of atherosclerosis by reducing both LDL-cholesterol and inflammation. The use of statin medications to treat coronary artery disease is a rational evidence-based treatment.

Effects of Coronary Artery Disease

With increased activity such as walking fast or running, the heart must beat faster to carry more oxygen to the exercising muscles. If a vessel is narrowed but not fully blocked, blood flow becomes inadequate during high need periods. The narrowing is a gradual change, so people may not recognize a difference. They just slow down or give up activities without realizing early fatigue is related to heart disease.

If the heart cannot respond to increased need because the inside diameter of the vessel is too small to carry adequate blood, the heart reacts to the lack of oxygen and discomfort occurs. *Angina* is chest pain caused by *ischemia,* lack of oxygen to the heart. When chest pain develops with increased activity and resolves with rest, it is called *exertional angina.* This is an important warning sign. If you experience exertional angina, see a doctor immediately for a full evaluation.

Sometimes the rough surface on a cholesterol plaque triggers the accumulation of blood clotting mediators. Platelets are the first step in the clotting mechanism. Floating in the blood, platelets stick to the rough area on the plaque and begin producing a clot. As the clot enlarges, the vessel closes.

Aspirin is a platelet inhibitor that interferes with the clotting process and helps keep the blood flowing. A daily low-dose aspirin, 81 mg, is of proven value in reducing clotting and preventing heart attacks. However, studies show chewing an aspirin before swallowing it works the fastest and is preferable in an emergency setting. Effects were seen within five minutes.

What Changes Should We Make?

Just as we have found in adults, overweight children as young as five years of age begin developing the same metabolic disorders as adults. To reduce cardiovascular disease in our nation and around the world in developed countries, early intervention is essential. We have the information, now all we need to do is make the right choices. Two prime actions are eating less fat and normalizing weight.

There is a global rise in child obesity. We think of the Japanese people as healthy and they are. Although incidence of childhood obesity is low, their rate has doubled in the past two decades. Recent news reports revealed an impressive change in Japanese school lunches is making headway to change this sudden rise in obesity. An improved school menu dominated by fresh ingredients, vegetables, soups, fish and rice has become Japanese policy. Children participate in both lunch preparation and serving as part of their education. They are served identical meals. Vending machines are barred from schools and the children are not allowed to bring food from home. Under this new policy, obesity in Japanese children has decreased in all ages, except for a consistent rise in late teens.

Here, the National School Lunch Act and the Child Nutrition Act provide the authority for the United States Department of Agriculture to govern school cafeteria food service. Over the course of a week, school meals must provide one-third or more of the daily nutrient needs. New standards for healthier school meals focus on avoiding fat, salt and sweets, substituting healthy fruits, vegetables and low-fat milk. Unfortunately, US meals still include high fat choices like pizza and French fries.

From many studies, we know coronary artery disease is pervasive in our society and begins in childhood where poor food choices and lack of exercise play a huge role. A recent study analyzed the relationships between fat metabolism, blood pressure and insulin resistance in 6-8 year-olds. The ability of arteries to expand and recoil, and their level of stiffness are predictors for atherosclerosis and the development of heart and arterial disease. In this scientifically important study, researchers found young children had already developed mild artery stiffness leading to impaired vascular health. Researchers stress the importance of lifestyle improvements beginning in childhood to include healthy food choices and exercise.

The Bogalusa Heart Study conducted over 30 years produced the largest information base of the natural history of cardiovascular risk factors, early heart disease, diabetes and hypertension in both Black and Caucasian populations. They found anatomic changes occurring in five to eight year old children, leading later to adult heart disease, atherosclerosis, coronary heart disease and hypertension. Environmental factors like smoking, exercise and diet significantly influence high cholesterol, high blood pressure and obesity. Many of these factors are directly controllable.

Lifestyles learned in early childhood play a strong role throughout life. Numerous programs have been developed to educate children about the importance of a healthy diet and exercise. Stemming from the Bogalusa study, numerous education modules are available.

Health Ahead/Heart Smart is one program for elementary children. The SuperKids SuperFit physical education program attempts to instill the concept of regular physical activity throughout life. Also available are educational modules for nutrition education and Family Health Promotion. Publications to promote healthy school lunches, noncompetitive physical education classes, health education curriculum materials, and many others are available from the Tulane University in New Orleans, tulane.edu/som/cardiohealth/materials.cfm at Tulane Center for Cardiovascular Health.

Starting healthy behaviors in childhood could play a large role in reducing health risks. If we start kids on an active lifestyle when they are young, the active behaviors often extend into adulthood. Kids need sixty minutes a day of vigorous activity five days a week combined with healthy eating. Coronary artery disease begins in obese sedentary children. Encouraging activity at a young age is beneficial in improving chances for a child's longevity. Energized by Michelle Obama, the "Let's Move!" campaign encourages kids to be active. In association with this program, to improve awareness and enthusiasm in children, many sports stars are engaging with kids to set examples and encourage them to be physically active.

Awareness, determination and goal-setting are all required to prevent cardiovascular disease. Much is known about healthy eating and behaviors. Research is ongoing and in time, preventing cardiovascular disease will become easier. Over the years of intensive research in this field, many factors contributing to the development of coronary artery disease have surfaced. We have control over most of them.

Most importantly, researchers have found a correlation between genetic links to inflammation and a predisposition to heart disease. Some inherited genetic mutations are linked to two of the most important risk factors in heart disease, LDL cholesterol and high blood pressure. Our hope is that researchers will find an inexpensive way to genetically "fingerprint" factors so each one can be addressed before the disease begins. This research phase is in its infancy now so it will be years before we have the ability to stop atherosclerosis entirely. In the meantime, there are many actions to take now that will make a positive difference.

Chapter 3
Risk Factors for Coronary Artery Disease

Why is coronary artery disease the leading cause of death?

Atherosclerosis is a disease of affluence. In developed countries throughout the world where food is plentiful, coronary artery disease is the leading cause of death. We eat, not only because we feel hungry, we eat to pass time, we eat for enjoyment, and we munch mindlessly at social events. The fact is, we eat too much and it's making us sick.

Coronary artery disease is tied to obesity. Food choices, portion sizes and exercise interplay, but the disease is more complex than any of these factors.

Statistics are boring to read and don't mean much when they are without a face. But consider the fact that 50% of all people have high blood pressure, high cholesterol or smoke; all three factors cause heart disease. Many of us personally know someone with these problems. Is it you? A loved one? You have the ability to make healthy choices and improve your health by treating these factors.

Part of the high death rate from heart disease is due to a lack of education about the cause and what can be done to fight it. But even knowing sound health practices, many people do not follow them. In recent years, there has been a reduction in heart deaths through improved treatment, education and reduction of risk factors, but coronary artery disease still remains the leading cause of death.

Two programs to address education, diagnosis and treatment are: the *Million Hearts* initiative, developed by the Department of Health and Human Services, with a goal to prevent a million heart attacks and strokes by 2017; and the *WISEWOMAN* program, administered through the Centers for Disease Control and Prevention.

Heart disease is a huge problem in developed countries around the world, including the United States. The *Million Hearts* program joined with the US Centers for Disease Control and Prevention, the American Heart Association and other organizations. Together they share strategies to reduce heart risk factors and save lives. Information from these organizations is available for education programs to implement change.

Your Heart

At 21 US sites, the *WISEWOMAN* project provides a screening and evaluation program to help women obtain healthcare when they have little or no insurance. Examinations, laboratory tests and education to lower risks are included.

Diabetes, overweight, poor diet choices, low physical activity and excess alcohol are all issues placing people at risk. If any of these affect you, take control, read more, learn more and make heart healthy changes. Don't become a statistic. Take action. Choose to reduce your personal risk factors.

According to the US Centers for Disease Control and Prevention, **50% of men and 64% of women who die suddenly of coronary heart disease have no previous symptoms**. Even if you have no symptoms, you may still be at risk for heart disease.

Katie, a registered nurse who believed she was healthy, working full time in a hospital but having difficulty with an arthritic knee finally decided to see an orthopedist. He recommended a total knee replacement procedure. As part of her preoperative evaluation, her primary physician evaluated her and performed an electrocardiogram. The electrical tracing of her heart conduction and rhythm was abnormal, indicating ischemia. A special nuclear medicine test of her heart showed marked reduction of circulation in the heart muscle. Katie went directly to the heart cath lab where two main coronary arteries were found to be more than 90% blocked by cholesterol plaques. The cardiologist dilated and stented both arteries. The orthopedic surgery had to be placed on hold. — Katie denies ever having any symptoms related to her heart.

Many people are aware that high cholesterol is associated with heart attacks, yet have never had a cholesterol blood test done. Because they have no symptoms, they can't believe they might be a candidate for a heart attack. The more you know how lifestyle, food choices and heredity factors impact heart health, the more equipped you will be to make healthy choices and obtain proper healthcare. This section provides more information on risk factors.

Risk Factor #1 – Tobacco Use
♥ **What to do**: Stop using tobacco and avoid second hand smoke.

Smoking dramatically increases heart attack risk and it is also the leading cause of cancer deaths in both men and women. Even if cholesterol levels are favorable, if you smoke, you are much more likely to have a heart attack than someone who does not smoke. The risk rises with the number of cigarettes smoked. All low-tar-cigarette, pipe and cigar smokers are at risk, too. If you have had a heart attack or stroke and continue to smoke, the risk for another cardiovascular event rises and life expectancy decreases.

Many people do not realize the significant harm *secondhand smokers* sustain. Coronary artery disease and lung cancer are directly linked to secondhand smoke.

Around the world, about 5 million people die each year from tobacco use. Medical practitioners everywhere agree smoking is harmful for both lungs and arteries throughout the body.

About 20% of people under the age of 65 are cigarette smokers while only 8% of those who are above that age smoke. Sixteen-percent of high school students smoke and about half that number use smokeless tobacco. Currently cigarettes cost about $5 per pack. Smoking one pack/day costs $150 a month. Not only is it a costly habit when it comes to health, it is a financial expense few can afford.

If you smoke or use tobacco in any way — quit. Don't start. If you are with anyone who smokes, do not allow them to smoke around you or your children. Heed a warning issued by the US Secretary of Health and Human Services: *Secondhand smoke is harmful and hazardous to the health of the general public and particularly dangerous to children. Inhaling secondhand smoke causes lung cancer and coronary heart disease in nonsmoking adults.*

Ventilated smoking areas and smoking in cars with the windows lowered are ineffective. Children exposed to secondhand smoke miss more school, have more breathing problems, asthma and ear infections than those without smoke exposure. Many states have banned smoking in cars when children are present. Because so many children and other nonsmokers are exposed to secondhand smoke around the world, the World Health Organization has orchestrated the creation of smoke-free environments.

Sudden infant death syndrome can be related to smoking. Autopsy findings commonly show elevated levels of nicotine and related substances in the baby's blood. In pregnant women who smoke, there is evidence of reduced fetal lung growth and a tendency to have low birth weight infants.

The National Cancer Institute reports the following cancers are tobacco-related: mouth, nasal cavity, throat, lung, esophagus, stomach, pancreas, kidney, bladder, cervix and acute myeloid leukemia. Using *smokeless tobacco* avoids the impact of smoke on the lungs, but vascular disease is increased, as are these many forms of cancer.

State and national campaigns provide help for people to stop smoking. Ask your healthcare provider if you need help to quit. The sooner you stop smoking or using any form of tobacco, the sooner your risks improve. The more you smoke and the longer you smoke, the higher your risk for vascular disease. Quitting lowers that risk. **Within 15 years of quitting, vascular risks from smoking drop to that of a non-smoker.** Studies show those who quit smoking after having a heart attack or stroke do much better than those who continue to smoke.

The arteries don't have a chance when the negative effects of smoking or secondhand smoke are combined with high blood pressure and high cholesterol.

From the National Institutes of Health the following information is validated by studies:

- Smoking alone doubles the risk for developing heart and artery disease.
- Combined with one additional risk factor, the risk of developing heart disease is 4 times higher; with two additional risk factors the estimated risk is increased by 8 times than for someone without risk factors.
- Sudden cardiac death is higher in smokers.
- Cigarette smoke contains nicotine, carbon monoxide, oxidant gases, particulate matter, carcinogenic hydrocarbons and other substances contributing to artery disease.

- Nicotine is a stimulant, raising heart rate and blood pressure.
- Carbon monoxide binds to red blood cells and blocks hemoglobin from carrying oxygen.
- Oxidizing chemicals in smoke reduce antioxidant levels and contribute to inflammation, cancers and other abnormalities including arterial damage and platelet activation that increases blood clotting.
- A high level of *acrolein* is found in smoke. This reactive substance causes many harmful effects at the cellular level that contribute to artery disease.

Noted in the information above, smoking, exposure to secondhand smoke and the use of smokeless tobacco are all dangerous and ought to be avoided. New laws restricting smoking in public places are important health actions.

Risk Factor #2 – High Blood Pressure
♥ **What to do**: Lower your blood pressure to a normal range.

Blood pressure is the force of blood against the walls of the arteries. High blood pressure puts stress on the heart and arteries. If the pressure inside the arteries is consistently above normal, it is known as high blood pressure or *hypertension*. High blood pressure is the most common form of cardiovascular disease and a leading cause of stroke and heart attacks. If hypertension is uncontrolled, it seriously increases your risk for heart disease, stroke, kidney disease, stroke-related blindness and dementia.

Blood pressure readings include two numbers – the upper number is called the *systolic*. The systolic reading is when the heart contracts and pushes blood out of the heart. The bottom number is called the *diastolic*. The diastolic reading is when the heart relaxes and fills with blood. The **American Heart Association** notes three levels to determine if your blood pressure is in a normal range, a pre-hypertension range, or hypertension range.

Numbers below identify blood pressure classifications:
Normal blood pressure: less than 120/80 mm/Hg
Pre-hypertension: 120 to 139/80 to 89 mm/Hg
Stage 1 Hypertension: 140 to 159/90 to 99 mm/Hg

Your Heart

Stage 2 Hypertension: 160+/100+ mmHg

In 2013 guidelines from the **American Diabetes Association** the target systolic blood pressure is **below 140 mmHg**. A large meta-analysis revealed no evidence that more stringent blood pressure control decreased heart attacks or death. These guidelines are published on an annual basis and may change in the future.

Many studies show a link between increased alcohol consumption and high blood pressure. Drinking more than 2 alcohol drinks/day for men, or 1/day for women, raises blood pressure. The actual mechanism is unclear and may have numerous causes. Acceleration of heart rate occurs as alcohol in the blood is metabolized by the liver reducing its sedating effects. Another powerful factor related to excess alcohol is sleep disturbance.

Some people use alcohol as a sedative to help them sleep, but the opposite actually happens. Alcohol interrupts normal sleep cycles, and can worsen sleep apnea. Sleep loss raises stress and reduces immunity. Chronic lack of sleep elevates blood pressure, heart rate and glucose levels, in addition to raising risk of stroke. Sleep specialists advise against a bedtime alcoholic beverage.

Between 25 to 30% of the adult US population have hypertension. Factors affecting blood pressure are age, weight, diet, lack of exercise, excess alcohol, smoking, race and family history. High blood pressure is often referred to as "the silent killer" because a person can have high blood pressure without having any symptoms.

Weight loss and exercise lower blood pressure, as do meditation and relaxation techniques. However, if you have hypertension, commonly called *essential hypertension* when there is no identifiable cause, all of the lifestyle changes you employ may not be adequate and you will need medication to bring it under control. If both of your parents have hypertension, you and your siblings will likely develop it, too. Hypertension is common in African-Americans who often develop the problem at a younger age than others.

What to do:
♥ It is important to know your numbers and take corrective action. Take control of your health.

- Purchase a blood pressure device.
- At first, check your blood pressure twice daily.
- Record the readings.
- Consult a doctor if the average reading is above 120/80 (or above 140 - if you choose to follow the American Diabetic Association guidelines).
- Bring your blood pressure device with you the next time you visit your health clinic and ask a medical practitioner to validate it for accuracy.

Do not be alarmed by occasional high pressure levels as readings fluctuate depending on activity and your stress state. There also may be malfunctions with your measuring equipment. It is important to follow instructions. Repeatedly checking a blood pressure alters blood flow in the arm and produces erroneous readings. Once your pressure is controlled and stable, monitor it at least weekly.

Look carefully at your average numbers. Even the pre-hypertension range places you at risk for heart disease and stroke. **The American Heart Association recommended goal is 120/80 or less.** Each year guidelines for control are released by various groups, so be sure to monitor health news for changes in recommendations.

Risk Factor #3 – High Blood Lipids (Cholesterol)
♥ **What to do:** Measure a lipid panel and treat as appropriate.

Cholesterol is composed of a variety of lipids (fats). Lipids are essential components of many body processes such as cell structure, hormones and fat storage for energy. Too much fat can be bad, causing a buildup of waxy fat within the walls of arteries. This process is first seen as fatty streaks in arteries can begin in childhood. Even elementary school children with lipid disorders and obesity show these changes.

Elevated cholesterol blood levels increase risk for cardiovascular disease and strokes. Obesity and the amount of saturated fat we eat contribute to the lipid levels. Genetics also play a large role in cholesterol metabolism and cardiovascular disease.

Triglycerides are in two basic forms, one of them transported in the blood, the other is all that adipose (fat) tissue stored throughout the body as an energy reserve. When you eat, the body converts unneeded calories into triglycerides and stores them in fat cells. If you regularly eat more calories than you burn, especially calories from carbohydrates and fats, you may have high triglycerides. When in excess, high triglycerides in the blood lead to coronary artery disease.

Fortunately, dietary changes and weight loss can help reduce triglycerides, but medications may also be necessary.

Two types of lipids discussed most frequently are the "good" and the "bad." The good High Density Lipoprotein (HDL) cholesterol helps carry the bad Low Density Lipoprotein (LDL) cholesterol away from plaques. The bad LDL cholesterol clogs arteries.

- Think of HDL as the "healthy" cholesterol – the number you want to be high. H=High
- Think of LDL as the "lard" – the number you want to be low. L=Low
- You want your HDL high and all other blood fats low.

Normal Blood Lipid Levels:

Total Cholesterol: 200 mg/dL or below

LDL: 100 to 129 mg/dL

If you have coronary artery disease or have had a heart attack, the LDL goal is lower: 70 mg/dL

HDL: 60 mg/dL or higher

Higher HDL numbers are considered best. HDL needs improvement if it is below 40 mg/dL in men or below 50 mg/dL in women

Triglyceride: 150 mg/dL or below

To measure common cholesterol components, a lipid test is done. Often the blood is drawn after fasting when you have had no food or drink for 12 hours. The only lipid test sensitive to eating is the triglyceride and you must be fasting to obtain an accurate number. Many additional lipid measurements may be ordered by specialists, on follow-up evaluations or in a research setting.

Risk Factor #4-Obesity, Diabetes and Metabolic Syndrome
♥ **What to do:** Normalize weight and blood glucose.

The discussion of obesity and diabetes are combined because excess weight places a person at serious risk for developing Type 2 diabetes and accelerated vascular disease.

Obesity and diabetes are now recognized as inflammatory diseases. Researchers have long found a correlation between inflammation and fatal cardiovascular disease. Obese people also tend to have high blood pressure, high cholesterol and diabetes — all serious risks for heart attack and stroke.

Over one-third of all adults living in the United States are obese. Both adult and childhood obesity have become problematic throughout our society. Many obese adults develop periodic blood glucose (sugar) elevations consistent with the pre-diabetic state of glucose intolerance. At that point, **weight loss may normalize blood glucose**, but monitoring is very important to assure there is no recurrence. Without interventions such as weight loss and increased activity, usually **within ten years the periodic blood glucose elevations evolve to the persistent high blood glucose levels of Type 2 diabetes**. It is important to avoid diabetes as long as possible.

If you have diabetes, you are more likely to:
- Develop high blood lipid levels including triglycerides and LDL-cholesterol.
- Die of heart disease and stroke than someone without diabetes.

♥ The Diabetes Prevention Program research project found weight loss by dietary changes combined with either increased activity, or with the diabetic drug glucophage (Metformin), **could prevent or delay the onset of Type 2 diabetes.** All people in the study were in the prediabetic state. Those who lost weight and exercised reduced their risk by 58%. Those taking the medication glucophage reduced their risk by 31%. **This information is extremely important because it shows you can make changes to substantially improve health, ward off Type 2 diabetes and reduce the risk for vascular disease. Prediabetics are encouraged to discuss lifestyle modification guidelines and use of glucophage with a health practitioner.**

Your Heart

Obesity and Metabolic Syndrome

Type 2 diabetes, affecting over 20 million people in the US, is related to the epidemic of obesity and another disorder occurring when body fat accumulates around the waist line. This is *metabolic syndrome*. In metabolic syndrome high blood glucose, high blood pressure, high cholesterol and insulin resistance occur. The first step in treatment is not drugs — it is weight loss, just like it is in lowering triglycerides.

It is believed that *insulin resistance* leading to diabetes is due to chronic low grade inflammation in fat tissues. A very important animal study just released in April 2013, also links the epidemic of diabetes and heart disease with inflammation and obesity-triggered autoimmune diseases that occur when the body generates antibodies against itself. The actual mechanism for this response is unknown.

In Type 2 diabetes, tissue cells are resistant to insulin. Even though there is an **increased insulin level** in the blood, in time, oral medications combined with calorie restriction are inadequate to control blood glucose. Insulin is essential for glucose to enter cells and be utilized for energy so Type 2 diabetics often evolve to requiring injections of the hormone insulin.

In Type 1 diabetes there is **inadequate insulin** production by the pancreas. The deficiency must be treated with insulin injections. Pills to lower blood glucose are not adequate even when combined with proper eating because the cells that produce insulin have been destroyed. Blood glucose must be monitored using capillary blood, eating must be controlled and Type 1 diabetics must inject insulin to normalize blood glucose levels.

What about *belly fat?* Abdominal obesity is the topic of many television and Internet ads touting methods to rid the body of belly fat. — The esthetic desire to look thinner is their focus, not targeting the intra-abdominal fat known as *visceral fat* — the fat that surrounds internal organs. The two fat compartments are: subcutaneous fat (the layer just under the skin) and intra-abdominal fat (the fat that packs itself around the heart, intestines and other abdominal organs). Fat in both areas are of medical concern because of related health risks.

For most people, losing weight is not easy. A later section describes an effective method of weight loss using marked calorie restriction for two days each week coupled with eating healthy low-fat meals for five days. This method reduces insulin resistance and improves blood glucose control. Our next Lipstick Logic Health Series book topic is obesity. It will address current research advances, weight control measures and the health benefits of weight loss.

Sometimes years before a person is aware of the problem, prediabetes with *insulin resistance* begins to develop. With prediabetes there are obvious markers. If the diagnosis is made early, the progression toward Type 2 diabetes can be interrupted, delayed or prevented. These markers include: obesity, a large waist, high triglycerides, high blood pressure, elevated blood glucose and a low HDL. Thoughtful calorie reduction, carbohydrate restriction, weight loss and exercise are all actions to reduce risk factors leading to heart disease and Type 2 diabetes.

Insulin resistance means muscle, liver cells and other cells don't respond to normal levels of insulin so blood glucose rises. The pancreas then produces more insulin to compensate; this is the evolution to Type 2 diabetes. Most obese people with excess stores of fat around the waist become insulin resistant and develop Type 2 diabetes. However, you do not have to be overweight to develop Type 2 diabetes.

An interesting finding in ongoing studies shows a person can be thin and still have excess visceral fat that correlates with insulin resistance, also placing them at increased risk for atherosclerosis.

Metabolically active visceral fat releases harmful substances that increase inflammation, blood clotting, blood pressure and reduce insulin sensitivity. In addition, harmful higher LDL, the bad cholesterol, and lower HDL, the good cholesterol, together are correlated with intra-abdominal fat accumulation.

♥ **What to do about abdominal fat**:
- Weight loss results in reduction of fat everywhere, including intra-abdominal fat.
- Eat smaller portions. Eat whole grains, fresh fruits and produce. Eat Mediterranean.
- Avoid fat and all fried food.

Your Heart

- Moderate exercise — 30-60 minutes per day if approved by your health practitioner.
- Strength training may be helpful.

Note: Doing sit-ups and spot exercising tightens muscles but does not change visceral fat.

Look AHEAD (Action for Health in Diabetes) is a US study supported by the National Institutes of Health involving 5,000 overweight or obese Type 2 diabetics from sixteen health centers. Participants were placed into one of two programs:
- General diabetes education related to food choices and exercise (the control group) –or–
- Intensive lifestyle intervention for Type 2 diabetics

After 9.6 years, the trial was stopped in September 2012. In the control group, there was gradual consistent weight loss. But of most importance, **there was no reduction in cardiovascular events in the intensive lifestyle intervention group**. Lifestyle interventions included healthy food choices, exercise and weight loss along with normalizing blood glucose.

The intensive lifestyle group had more initial weight loss but regained some, both groups ended with weight reduction. Both groups showed health benefits with improved glucose control and reduction of cardiovascular risk factors. In addition, the intensive group had fewer hospitalizations, less medication, less kidney disease, lower retinopathy (diabetic eye changes) and lower incidence of depression. However, diet and exercise provided no measurable protection against heart disease for these diabetics.

Cardiovascular risks rise with the duration of diabetes so prevention is important. Once diabetes develops, it remains important to exercise, eat a healthy diet and practice self glucose management to reduce kidney and visual impairment.

Diabetics must learn how to eat to avoid glucose elevation. "Feeling" when the glucose is high does not work. Diabetics must take control of their health and measure their glucose levels by capillary blood checks. Guessing is not good enough because risks rise with blood glucose elevation and duration.

Betty Kuffel, MD

Remember, any food you eat can be stored as fat. Even red wine, touted to raise HDL which we want high, should be used in moderation. Unfortunately, alcohol also raises triglycerides, adds calories and carries other risks.

How do you know if your weight places you at higher risk for heart disease?
A measurement called the Body Mass Index (BMI) is used to estimate a person's body fat. Not everyone agrees the BMI is an accurate reflection of fatness, but at minimum, it is an excellent screening tool. Some say all you need to do is measure your waist. Abdominal obesity correlates highly with heart disease risk. A large University of Bristol and Copenhagen University Hospital study of 76,000 people found for every 8.8 pounds increase in weight, there was a 52% increase in risk for developing coronary heart disease.

To emphasize the important relationship of obesity to heart disease, findings presented at the annual meeting of the European Society of Cardiology in 2012 included a study on nearly 100 adolescents who had no symptoms of heart disease. Yet, they had hearts showing evidence of damage with thicker walls and functional impairment.

♥ Check Your Waist Size to Screen for Obesity:
If your fat is predominantly around your waist and not around your hips, you are at higher risk for both heart disease and Type 2 diabetes. To properly measure your waist, stand upright, place a tape measure around your mid-section just above the hip bones, exhale and read the measurement. In women, a waist size greater than 35 inches correlates with increased risk. In men, a waist size of 40 inches or higher correlates with increased risk.

Use Body Mass Index (BMI) to screen for obesity:
Values for BMI set at a National Institutes of Health consensus conference are:
BMI of less than 18.5 indicates you are thin.
BMI between 18.6 and 24.9 indicates you are at a healthy weight.
BMI between 25 and 29.9 indicates you are overweight.
BMI of 30 or greater indicates obesity.

Your Heart

♥ How to determine your BMI number:
1. Weigh yourself on a reliable scale. Let's say you weigh 140 pounds.
2. Measure your height. Let's say you are 5 feet 3 inches or 63 inches tall.
3. Multiply your height x your height. (Example: 63 in. x 63 in. = 3969 inches)
4. Divide your weight in pounds by your height x your height and multiply the total x 703. (Example = 24.8)

Or, go to: http://www.nhlbi.nih.gov/guidelines/obesity/ BMI/bmicalc.htm and use the National Institutes of Health online BMI calculator. Just fill in your numbers and it will calculate your BMI.

United States weight statistics compiled in 2012 show: 77% of all adult men and 59% of all adult women, of all nationalities, are overweight and about 30% of them are obese. Colorado has the lowest number of obese people at 18%. West Virginia has the highest at 35.3%. **Food choices make a difference.**

In an extensive study involving 175 countries analyzing diabetes and its relationship to nutrition, researchers found sugar availability correlated directly with diabetes prevalence. When degree of sugar exposure and duration dropped, so did diabetes. In addition, they analyzed factors related to diabetes such as exercise and obesity. Diabetes incidence was not explained by activity or excess weight.

Another study, supporting findings related to sugar intake, examined more than 12,000 people with Type 2 diabetes, comparing them with over 16,000 people without diabetes. **Researchers found the risk of developing Type 2 diabetes rose 22% by drinking one 12-ounce sugar-sweetened soft drink per day.**

A French study involving 66,000 people examined the relationship between diet soda and diabetes. They found an intake of **20 ounces of diet soda per week also correlated with increased Type 2 diabetes**. There is no proven causative link but based on all of these studies, what should we do? **Drink water. Avoid both sweetened and sugar-free drinks. If you like flavoring, add a slice of citrus, cucumber or a bit of fresh mint to your water.**

31

Elevated blood sugar accelerates the development of coronary artery disease in all ages. The same disease processes occur in children as in adults. Type 2 diabetes was previously considered an older person's disease. Now it is occurring in childhood. Their blood glucose rises. Type 2 diabetes occurs and arteries narrow.

♥ Each family could begin a path to better health by changing daily activities and foods. Choices to improve health:
- Eliminate all fried foods including chips.
- Eliminate sugared and diet drinks.
- Limit sugary snacks, sugared breakfast cereals and carbohydrates like bread and crackers.
- Eat rice or pasta only twice a week.
- Substitute fresh fruit and veggies such as carrots and peapods for processed snacks.

People who have either Type 1 or Type 2 diabetes are at increased risk for developing both heart and arterial disease. Glucose elevations, inflammation, and lipid elevations occur in both diseases. This damages heart arteries and extends throughout the aorta, abdominal and leg arteries. Normalizing blood glucose and lipids decreases risk for coronary vascular disease along with related kidney disease and blindness.

Coronary artery bypass surgery and angioplasty procedures to open arteries are more successful in non-diabetics than in diabetics. To prolong life and decrease disease advancement, a healthy lifestyle is essential. Healthful eating and exercising daily both help to normalize blood glucose levels.

Goals in non-diabetics: blood pressure below 120/80, normal lipid levels.

Note: American Diabetic Association 2013 guidelines recommend a systolic blood pressure below 140 and not below 120 because a large study did not show the lower blood pressure reduced heart attacks or deaths. However, along with the blood pressure below 140, it is important to follow additional standardized goals: normalize lipids, glucose control based on self-measurement, decrease risk of kidney failure by taking an ACE inhibitor medication to reduce protein loss from the kidneys.

Obesity impacts pregnancy. Inactive, obese and smoking women are more likely to have complicated pregnancies with risks to both the mother and infant. Some conditions occurring during pregnancy correlate with the later development of related health problems. These include: *preeclampsia* (accelerated high blood pressure sometimes requiring bed rest or even C-section delivery), *gestational diabetes* (when blood sugars rise in pregnant women due to the stress of pregnancy), and *pregnancy-induced-hypertension*.

Gestational diabetics often give birth to large babies weighing ten pounds and more. These large babies, surprisingly, are not as strong and resilient as smaller newborns. Large, premature or under-weight babies are prone to low blood glucose levels.

A study revealed babies born to overweight or obese mothers already had arterial wall thickening, an early sign of artery disease. With this finding, the concern is — will these babies born to overweight mothers go on to have increased risk of early heart and vascular disease?

Maternal glucose levels typically respond favorably following childbirth. If there was significant weight gain during the pregnancy, it is very important to lose the weight and monitor capillary glucose levels to assure a quick return to normal glucose levels through diet, exercise and medication. Gestational diabetes raises the likelihood of developing Type 2 diabetes later in life.

Blood pressure monitoring and treatment during pregnancy are high priorities. Serious issues related to elevated blood pressure during pregnancy are fetal complications with preterm delivery and related fetal or infant deaths. Women with high blood pressure during pregnancy are also more apt to develop hypertension and heart disease requiring treatment.

Results of numerous studies show the most common cause of maternal death is heart disease. Three million women age 18-44 have heart disease including about 1% of pregnant women. Researchers note maternal cardiac deaths are due to many factors. Heart attacks in pregnant women may have increased in recent years because more women are delaying

Betty Kuffel, MD

pregnancies. The women are older. Pregnancy causes the heart to work harder, beat faster, and handle a higher blood volume load. At an older age, some women are less physically active, have developed diabetes and have higher lipid levels placing them at higher risk for coronary artery disease and heart stress. Pregnancy is a natural process but is not without risk.

Risk Factor #5 – Physical Inactivity
♥ **What to do:** Exercise regularly, 30-60 minutes/day.

Inactivity contributes to poor health. Exercise is highly correlated with health and longevity. Sitting at a computer writing for hours, watching television, or reading without taking breaks to exercise, are all examples of spending too much time in a chair.

We all know exercise is good for us and yet television watching is a common pastime. Numerous studies show the sedentary behavior of watching television actually shortens life. In a US study, for every two hours spent each day watching television, the risks of cardiovascular disease and diabetes rise. Part of this is related to unhealthy eating coupled with long periods sitting.

If you watch TV or perform other prolonged sedentary tasks such as long-haul trucking or driving for prolonged periods, take periodic walks and avoid caloric snacks. At home, even better, place your treadmill or stationary bicycle in front of the screen. Exercise while you watch and lower your heart risks.

A sedentary lifestyle impacts health at any age. It is very important to make regular exercise part of your life. Before starting an exercise program, especially if you have underlying medical problems, be sure to consult your healthcare provider for guidelines.

Remember to take a break. Get up and go for a walk, but return right here to learn more about the risks of cardiac disease and the measures you can take to prevent or begin reversing some of the negative effects of inactivity.

Risks Factor #6 – Eating the Wrong Foods
♥ **What to do:** Choose healthful foods and practice portion control. Consider following the Mediterranean diet.

34

Your Heart

You've probably heard the saying: "You are what you eat." Unfortunately, there is a lot of truth to that statement. Both easy-access and increased consumption of sugar correlate with an increase in obesity and diabetes. If you eat appropriate portion sizes of healthy foods like fruits and vegetables, fish like salmon, and other low-fat proteins, you probably have healthy arteries and your weight is not an issue. On the other hand, if you eat a diet high in carbohydrates, sugar and fat, your weight and arteries will provide telltale evidence.

The American Heart Association, recommends limiting daily sugar consumption to no more than 100 calories per day. Sugar adds non-nutritious calories leading to extra pounds and reduction in heart health.

Many foods, including bread, are complex carbohydrates the body converts to glucose. Sugar may also be added to bread. Be sure to read labels. One regular Oreo cookie packs 45 calories. The double-stuffed ones have 70 calories each. Oreo calories are primarily from sugar and fat. It's hard to eat just one Oreo. (For calorie comparison: One tablespoon of sugar granules = 45 calories.)

Salt consumption is another factor that increases your blood pressure and risk of coronary artery disease. A snack of 3-4 ounces of potato chips at 120 mg of sodium/ounce makes up about one-third of daily recommended intake of salt. Both the salt and fat content of chips make them a bad food choice. Baked chips are healthier and lower in fat, but eating an apple is much better for your health. Table salt is sodium chloride.

When you read labels, you will see sodium as an ingredient. The maximum salt or sodium allowable each day is 1500 mg. (For comparison: One 10 ¾ ounce can of regular Campbell's Tomato Soup contains 2.5 servings. Each ½ cup portion contains 90 calories and 480 mg of sodium.) One can nearly reaches the top daily allowable amount for an adult.

High salt and low potassium are both linked to high blood pressure. An analysis of 56 studies showed reducing sodium intake was associated with reduced blood pressure and a reduction in strokes and fatal heart attacks.

Another study analyzing data from 128,000 people revealed increasing dietary potassium lowered blood pressure in adults.

Reducing dietary salt and increasing foods rich in potassium will help normalize blood pressure and save lives. Because some people with kidney problems must limit both sodium and potassium, it is necessary to check with your physician before a diet change.

♥ To reduce salt/sodium in your diet, add no salt to your food, avoid processed meats and be sure to read labels so you know what you are consuming. Most canned soups are high in sodium. However many brands, including Campbell's, have heart healthy low sodium options. Try soups and canned vegetables that are low-sodium.

♥ To increase potassium in your diet, eat: oranges, melons, spinach, mushrooms, dried apricots, yogurt, salmon, avocados, potatoes, bananas and beans.

A diet high in saturated and trans fats will increase coronary artery disease risk. Take note of calories, fats, cholesterol, sugar and sodium by checking the "NUTRITIONAL FACTS" printed on package labels.

♥ The American Heart Association provides guidelines for the amount of sugar, salt, fat and cholesterol to include in your daily diet:
- Sugars — For women: no more than 24 grams/day (100 calories.
- Sugars — For men: 36 grams/day (150 calories).
- Salt — less than 1,500 mg of sodium/day.
- Saturated Fats — less than 7% of total daily calories. Fat equals 9 calories/gram. In a 2,000 calorie diet this would be 2000 x .07 = 140/9 =15 grams of fat.
- Trans Fat — maximum of 2 grams/day. Aim for zero.
- Cholesterol — less than 300 mg/day for a healthy adult.

Risk Factor #7 – Calcium
♥ **What to do:** Choose dietary calcium. Ask your physician about stopping calcium supplements.

Recent studies have shown increased risk for heart attacks in those taking supplements. Knowing what supplements to take or not to take isn't always easy. As more medical studies are completed and new information is learned, long-standing recommendations in many areas of health change.

Hip fractures and spine compression fractures are common in post menopausal women. For several years, physicians have measured bone density and advocated supplemental calcium and vitamin D to maintain bone strength.

When we speak of having healthy bones, this means the bone mineral density is normal. If the mineral density is below normal, there is evidence of weakening in the bone structure and *osteopenia* is present. If osteopenia worsens, bones become weaker, more porous and at risk for fracture. At that point the condition is called *osteoporosis*.

Calcium, vitamin D and additional medications thought to enhance bone strength are prescribed for those with marked bone loss. Based on the outcome of the following study, the practice of taking calcium supplements is changing. The next article is highlighted because it shows a **high intake of supplemental calcium is a risk factor for heart disease**.

In February 2013, a study examined calcium intake and cardiovascular health in more than 60,000 women. Over a 19 year period, nearly 4,000 women died from cardiovascular disease. **Death rates from heart disease and stroke doubled in women who consumed more than 1400 mg of calcium supplements a day, plus ate diets that included calcium, vs. women who consumed a total of 600-999 milligrams of calcium/day.** There is no proven cause and effect but this association appears hazardous.

This report is of importance because many older men and women take extra calcium supplements to prevent and treat bone loss. Many are taking the dosage risk level. Does that include you?

Also, women who to consumed <u>inadequate</u> amounts, less than 600 milligrams of calcium/day, also had a higher death rate.

Dr. Gregg Fonarow, cardiologist at UCLA and an American Heart Association spokesman, recommends calcium supplements be taken only if benefits to bone health outweigh the potential of cardiovascular disease risks. If you are taking a calcium supplement, please check with your physician to discuss whether your risk for bone disease outweighs the risk for cardiovascular disease.

Another large study published in February 2013, sponsored by the National Institutes of Health also examined calcium and heart disease. This study assessed over 300,000 men and women revealed **a high intake of calcium supplements in men increased heart risk**. Findings in this study, however, did not show the same risk in women.

The results of these two studies are disturbing because they contradict what many people have considered healthy — taking calcium supplements. Now, because of these findings, **some physicians advocate stopping calcium supplements.**

The human body tightly regulates the amount of calcium in the blood, but a high intake can override the body's natural controls. More large studies are needed to develop evidence-based guidelines. If you are currently taking calcium and vitamin D supplements, ask your physician for guidance. If you have osteoporosis or osteopenia, your management may change.

The latest recommendation from the U.S. Preventive Services Task Force: **A daily vitamin D supplement of more than 400 IU, and 1000 mg of calcium have no net benefit for primary prevention of fractures.**

This is a very important statement because the article reported that surveys show more than 50% of women over the age of 60 are taking supplements of both vitamin D and calcium. Osteoporosis affects 1 in 4 women and 1 in 8 men over the age of 50. So the question is: Are postmenopausal women who are taking supplements to enhance their health and make their bones strong unknowingly increasing their risk for heart disease and death? Men on calcium supplements may also be at risk.

Dairy products contain calcium, protein, phosphorous, magnesium, vitamin D and potassium. All of them are important elements in bone health. But, nutrition experts are not advocating cow's milk as a dietary source of calcium because there are healthier sources. For example, Asian populations, where milk consumption is low because of common lactose intolerance, have stronger bones and fewer hip fractures than their American counterparts. The Asian diet includes calcium-rich vegetables and common foods such as fish-cakes made from ground fish containing calcium from fish bones.

Okinawans have 40% fewer hip fractures than Americans. They have more sun exposure, daily physical activity and eat more high-calcium soy products. Even the drinking water on Okinawa contains minerals not found in most fresh water.

Other than moving to Okinawa and following their active lifestyle and diet, what can we do to achieve their state of health and longevity?

- Reduce our consumption of fatty milk products.
- Eat soy and other foods containing calcium.

Almond milk (non-sweetened) contains only 40 calories/cup. *Fortified* almond milk is a good source of calcium, plus 3 grams of fat but no saturated fat, 2 grams of carbohydrates and 1 gram of dietary fiber. (Eating almonds for calcium supplementation is not a good choice because of the calorie content. A whole cup of almonds contains 378 milligrams of calcium but 800 calories.) Additional products from non-dairy source are also worth trying. Coconut milk and many others of nut origin are tasty and healthful. Be sure to read the labels.

There are many ways to add calcium to your diet. The usual mantra is *milk builds strong bones.* But do adults need milk? The answer is no. There are nutritious aspects of milk, but it is important to examine the negative impact of milk products and fat consumption on heart health and make an informed choice.

Cheese is a nutritious protein and calcium source. However, cheese is high in calories and fat, and often high in sodium. **In the American diet, cheese is the highest source of saturated fat.** Eating cheese contributes to obesity and heart risks. Choose low-fat items if you choose to eat dairy products. Read labels and make your choices wisely.

For years we have consumed large amounts of milk, sometimes called "liquid meat." Cow's milk is nutritious containing proteins, vitamin D, phosphorous and calcium. All are needed for strong bones but milk also contains saturated fat and calories that could be spent elsewhere. Even drinking 3 cups of 2% milk per day adds 400 calories.

Many people cannot consume milk or milk products because their bodies do not produce the digestive enzyme *lactase*. Without *lactase* they cannot digest lactose, the sugar in milk. When lactase-deficient people drink milk and eat milk products, such as cottage cheese and ice cream, they develop abdominal discomfort, bloating and diarrhea. Other people are actually allergic to milk and must avoid all dairy products.

If you choose not to drink milk or do not tolerate it because of an allergy, lactose intolerance or because you are avoiding the animal fat and calories, there are many other dietary sources for calcium and the other nutrients found in milk.

♥ **Calcium** is found in broccoli, green leafy vegetables, fortified soy milk, tofu and baked beans. Tofu, a bean cake made from soy, is high in calcium. One-half cup of tofu made with calcium sulfate = 434 milligrams of dietary calcium.

♥ **Potassium** is found in many sources: oranges, melons, spinach, mushrooms, dried apricots, yogurt, salmon, avocados, potatoes, bananas, beans and other choices.

♥ **Magnesium** is in spinach, nuts, oatmeal, beans and halibut.

♥ **Phosphorus**-rich foods include fish, nuts, and cereals.

♥ As more information evolves on this topic, you will find news reports, and updates at YourHeartBook.com. In the meantime, if you already suffer from bone loss, follow your physician's instructions, but consider obtaining significant calcium from plant-based sources.

For calcium to be absorbed, adequate vitamin D must be consumed. This raises two other issues — how much vitamin D is enough and where do we get it?

Vitamin D is synthesized in the body by changing a form of cholesterol found in the skin, to *cholecalciferol* in a process requiring UV-B rays from sunlight. Cholecalciferol is the form of vitamin D3 the body uses. With so many people wearing sun blocker lotions to avoid sunburn, melanoma and other skin cancers, UV-B sun rays are blocked and less vitamin D is made by the body. As a result, vitamin D must be obtained in supplements or food.

As of 2011, the daily vitamin D_3 recommendation for adult women and men, ages 18-70 is 600 IU/day and above age

70 is 800 IU/day. Food sources of vitamin D include: fish such as salmon and tuna, and fortified breakfast cereals.

People living in Northern latitudes with little sun exposure have lower vitamin D levels. Doses for vitamin D remain controversial and should be discussed with your physician. Some people need much higher doses to reach a normal level. Vitamin D blood levels can be monitored and proper dosing recommended. Like all fat-soluble vitamins (A, D, E & K), it is possible to take too much and become vitamin-toxic. Vitamin D levels in the normal range correlate with heart health.

If you are concerned about bone health, weight-bearing exercise, such as walking, is clearly beneficial. Scientists at the University of Pennsylvania tracked the diets and exercise in females ages 12-18 and found the greatest gain in bone mass occurred in exercisers, (not those who ingested the most calcium). It is during the teen years that females actually gain most of their total bone mass. **Bone density relates highly to what occurred during the teenage years with exercise being most important.** However, calcium is important along with phosphorous, potassium and magnesium. They are required for many body processes including bone metabolism and strength.

Risk Factor #8 – Marijuana, Cocaine, Methamphetamine and MDPV

♥ **What to do:** Weigh benefits/risks of marijuana use. Do not use cocaine, methamphetamine or MDPV.

Marijuana

At an American Heart Association meeting, Murray A. Mittleman, MD, PhD, of Beth Israel Deaconess Hospital in Boston, reported a study showing a clear link between smoking marijuana and having a heart attack within one to two hours of lighting up. He stated marijuana smokers who had heart attacks related to marijuana smoking were younger with an average age of 44 and had fewer risk factors than nonsmokers, whose average age was 62. It is unknown if the negative effect on the heart is related to the drug or to a smoke component.

Marijuana contains many active substances but THC (delta-9-tetrahydrocannabinol) is the main psychoactive substance and is often referred to as *cannabis,* from the attractive flowering plant genus, including *Cannabis sativa* and others. Symptoms of marijuana use include: rapid heart rate, elevated blood pressure, increased respiratory rate, dry mouth, slow reaction time and red eyes. In addition, men who are heavy marijuana users may have a lower sperm count and lower testosterone levels.

There can be long term effects in those who smoke marijuana regularly. We know particulate matter contained in marijuana smoke carries health hazards, reduces lung function and damages airway mucus membranes. Similar to tobacco smoking, smoking marijuana may carry an increased risk for some forms of cancer. The drug is psychologically addictive with dependence rates higher in daily smokers. In young developing brains, negative aspects are seen.

Medical marijuana is used to help patients with many chronic conditions. Some of these are to:

- Reduce debilitating pain syndromes
- Help cancer patients by reducing nausea from chemotherapy
- Stimulate appetite, reduce pain and improve sleep in multiple sclerosis
- Improve quality of life for people with terminal illness

In a recent study, there were lower levels of fasting insulin and smaller waist circumference in marijuana users. The negative side effects must be weighed against beneficial effects. Compared to alcohol, marijuana is a benign drug. But, like alcohol and tobacco, frequent use can cause health problems.

Cocaine
Cocaine is a powerful addictive illicit drug in common use today. Users often take the drug in binges. To attain the desired effect, higher and higher doses are required. Cocaine use causes severe heart and blood vessel damage. Anyone who uses this addictive drug is at high risk for heart attack at any age. People in their 20s can die of the effects. If pregnant women take the drug, fetal damage is common. "Crack babies" born to mothers taking cocaine are at risk for major brain structure and neurologic, cognitive and behavior abnormalities.

Your Heart

Cocaine's profound effect on the brain produces hyperactivity in users resulting from increased activity of dopamine, a neurotransmitter. Users of cocaine may stay awake for days. Use correlates with strokes, memory loss and learning problems. A Harvard study showed vessel constriction in the brain occurs even with small amounts of cocaine.

After long periods of abstinence, the cocaine experience persists with intense craving. Relapse is common. Using cocaine sets you on a destructive life course leading to an addiction appearing to be as difficult to kick as methamphetamine. Both drugs affect dopamine function involving motivation, reward and pleasure. Numerous studies show brain areas involved in emotional response and craving may be permanently damaged.

Methamphetamine
Known as "crystal meth" or "meth" — this is a disastrous drug both physically and emotionally. Similar to cocaine in many ways, it is a highly addictive stimulant. Brain alteration in areas associated with memory and emotion occur no matter how is it used; whether snorted, smoked or injected. Its action is to increase the release and block the reuptake of the dopamine. When dopamine levels soar, intense euphoria occurs. Signs visible to observers include: users becoming talkative, aggressive, agitated, sometimes overly confident, and paranoid.

Brain effects include blood vessel spasms and inflammation that appear to weaken the arteries leading to rupture and bleeding. Seizures are common. The risk for *hemorrhagic stroke,* sudden bleeding in the brain, is five times higher in meth users than non-meth users.

Methamphetamine damages the brain, kidneys and lives. Heart and vascular risks are high. Use results in a rapid pulse, high blood pressure, eroded teeth, heart attacks, strokes and inflammation of the inside of the heart called *endocarditis.* Cardiac arrest sometimes occurs. Users at any age, even teenagers, are at risk for these problems.

MDPV (methylenedioxypyrovalerone)
Better known as "bath salts" on the street, this and other related synthetic stimulants are illicit drugs without medicinal

value and have a high potential for abuse. The Synthetic Drug Abuse Prevention Act makes it illegal to possess and distribute, and illegal to possess the chemicals for manufacture. Users snort, shoot or ingest the drugs to get high. In the process, they develop paranoia, sometimes suicidal thinking, hallucinations and agitation, along with chest pain, rapid heart rate and high blood pressure.

Your Heart

Chapter 4
Understanding Cholesterol

What is Cholesterol?

Cholesterol in the body consists of various forms of fat called lipids. These fat molecules are transported in the blood with protein carriers. Together, they are called *lipoproteins*. The lipoproteins are essential in body processes including cell structure, hormones and fat storage for energy. Many people have genetically faulty lipid transport systems and are at higher risk for early heart disease than others.

The amount of saturated fat from animal sources consumed in the diet contributes to cholesterol levels but, even becoming a vegetarian will not result in normal cholesterol levels in everyone. Those with inherited disorders of lipid transport and metabolism may need to reduce their consumption of saturated fat while also taking a lipid-lowering drug to achieve normal levels and reduce cardiovascular risks.

♥ Lipid Panel goals:

Total Cholesterol: 200 mg/dL or below

LDL: 100 to 129 mg/dL

If you have coronary artery disease or have had a heart attack, the LDL goal is lower: 70 mg/dL

HDL: 60 mg/dL or higher

Higher numbers are considered best. HDL needs improvement if below 40 mg/dL in men or below 50 mg/dL in women

Triglyceride: 150 mg/dL or below

Even if you have no evidence of heart disease, are not diabetic and have no other known risk factors for developing heart disease, it is important to measure your lipid levels. Familial lipid disorders are prevalent. If early vascular disease is common in your family, lipid blood levels should be done early in life, even before age twenty. Before age 40, everyone should know their numbers. A lipid panel is a standard blood test. If you have never had one, schedule an evaluation with your health practitioner soon.

Know your numbers and make changes to normalize them under the guidance of your healthcare provider.

Betty Kuffel, MD

Familial hypercholesterolemia causes very early ischemic heart disease. Even in childhood, signs of the disease are evident as yellow lesions on palms. If left untreated, fatty plaques develop over tendons and around the eyes. In the most severe form, those affected may not survive to age 30.

Anyone with unusually high cholesterol (For example: LDL of 300mg/dL, total cholesterol of 600 mg/dL, or triglyceride levels above 500 mg/dL), should be referred to a specialty lipid treatment center or endocrinologist for full evaluation and management. Sometimes the blood is purified by *aphaeresis*, a process that removes excess fat. Even an intestinal bypass may be done to reduce absorption of fat from the intestine to prolong life.

A young family, parents in their thirties and an 8 year old daughter, presented to my office for an evaluation for dietary counseling and weight reduction. The concerned parents were worried about their daughter's weight. The family resemblance was striking. Blond-haired, happy, talkative, and all heavy-set with large abdomens; the little girl weighed 100 pounds. Their family history included early death on both sides of the family. All grandparents died of sudden death or known heart attacks before age 60, some before age 40. History alone suggested an unfortunate genetic mix. All of them, even the little girl, had marked elevations of cholesterol and triglycerides. In fact, their blood in test tubes appeared rusty brown in color. After sitting a short time, a layer of fat rose to the surface — just like cream on fresh milk. I referred all of them to a specialist.

Unfortunately, if natural body processes go wrong, sometimes they go terribly wrong. Fat components begin accumulating within arteries even in childhood. As time goes by, the arteries become narrowed with waxy atherosclerosis. When an occlusion stops blood flow, oxygen transfer to tissues beyond the block is stopped. Without oxygen, that part of the heart muscle suffers a myocardial infarction and will die unless the block is cleared rapidly. In the heart, blood flow blockage causes a heart attack. In the brain, blood flow blockage causes a stroke. In a limb, unless the occlusion is removed, tissue dies and the limb must be amputated.

Your Heart

Each of these arterial closures is a devastating preventable problem. Thrombolytic clot-melting drugs or special invasive procedures may clear blockages. The artery can be enlarged and splinted open with a device called a stent, or may be bypassed. Permanent damage or death occurs unless blockages are rapidly cleared. Why wait until something happens? Take control now.

Even looking at the facial skin of some individuals, you can determine their heart risks.

For example, *Xanthelasma* is a condition where soft yellow plaques accumulate on the eyelid. *Xanth* is a Greek word for yellow and *elasma* means plate. These eyelid deposits are flat highly visible collections of foam cells filled with lipid material that have infiltrated the skin. Not everyone with this condition has high cholesterol, but the condition is an independent risk factor associated with heart disease and stroke. These skin lesions mirror changes occurring inside arteries.

In a European study involving 12,000 people over the age of thirty, those with visible xanthelasma also had more evidence of severe atherosclerosis and cardiovascular disease. So, if you have the flat yellow eyelid deposits of *xanthelasma,* even if your lipid panel is favorable, experts recommend drug treatment.

Good Cholesterol: High Density Lipoprotein (HDL)

A lipid profile usually provides a ratio of total cholesterol to HDL. Calculate your risk ratio by dividing the Total Cholesterol number by the HDL number. *Total Cholesterol/ HDL Ratio* is a good predictor of heart disease. The recommended ratio is 5 to 1 or lower.

A high HDL (the healthy, good one) correlates directly with a low risk of heart disease.

If your HDL number is low, this typically correlates with an increased risk of artery disease. To our benefit, researchers continue to look for ways to identify and improve risks. A high HDL is what we strive for and it usually correlates with a lower risk of heart disease.

Bad Cholesterol: Low Density Lipoprotein (LDL)

Remember the "L" in LDL as being lard or the lipid number you want low. What would happen to your kitchen plumbing if you were to pour bacon fat or melted lard down the drain? It would solidify and block the drain pipes. Food choices impact heart health. Eating a diet high in fat will clog arterial pipes by increasing LDL cholesterol accumulation within the arterial wall.

As the LDL rises, the risk for heart disease rises and the likelihood you will have a heart attack or stroke rises with it. As the HDL rises, the risk for heart disease falls. Lowering the LDL and raising the HDL helps to stop the disease process and is instrumental in reversing atherosclerosis.

Triglycerides

Hypertriglyceridemia is used to describe the health problem associated with elevated blood triglyceride. Components of the word make it easier to remember: *hyper* means high; *triglyceride* is the name of the fat; and *emia* means in the blood. You can have this disorder even when your total cholesterol is normal.

As explained earlier with the lard example, LDL collects inside arteries but it is important to note that *triglycerides collect everywhere* as stored energy, body fat. When calories are not processed or used for energy, they are stored in fat cells in the form of triglycerides, both as subcutaneous and intra-abdominal fat. Weight loss reduces both of the triglyceride stores, making you weigh less, and lowers blood triglyceride levels.

The body is very efficient in storing fat to be ready when food is scarce. Today food scarcity is not the problem it was in past centuries. With fast food restaurants located throughout America and unhealthy snacks sold in every grocery store, humans are exercising less and eating more fat, more sugar and more calories than they need. As a result, body-fat stores are accumulating at epidemic rates. Obesity has become a very visible and critical national health problem. There are many associated health issues including: disability due to the weight itself, joint damage, breathing difficulty, sleep apnea, diabetes, heart disease and increased risks for dementia.

Your Heart

<u>Medical problems correlated with high triglycerides</u>:

> Elevated blood sugars in both Type 1 and Type 2 diabetics
> Low thyroid hormone levels
> Obesity
> Chronic kidney failure
> Heavy alcohol consumption

The metabolic effects of alcohol on the liver and triglyceride levels have been known for years. The effect is not related to the type of alcohol; it is the same for beer, wine and hard liquor. However, the volume of consumption is important. Little effect is seen on triglyceride levels with moderate drinking: 1-3 glasses/day for men and 1-2 glasses for women. Alcohol abuse, especially in combination with obesity and diabetes, can result in severe hypertriglyceridemia. Levels may be as high as 1000 mg/dL and more! With this elevation, there is a high risk to develop pancreatitis. The serious inflammatory process in the pancreas often results in severe abdominal pain and hospitalization. Pancreatitis can be recurring and life-threatening.

<u>Numerous medications raise triglyceride levels</u>:

> Birth control pills
> Beta-blockers (lower heart rate and blood pressure)
> Diuretics (remove excess fluid)
> Steroids ex. prednisone (decrease inflammation)
> Tamoxifen (estrogen blocker used in breast cancer treatment)

Note: Many of these medications are essential, so triglyceride levels must be monitored and treated as necessary.

Cholesterol remnants

A recent Danish study showed a correlation between elevated triglycerides and another lipid sub-type called *cholesterol-remnant particles*. If you have elevated triglycerides and elevated cholesterol remnants, you are more likely to develop heart disease. Remnant particles have been studied for many years but are not usually tested except in research settings. A triglyceride level is measured on the standard lipid panel.

49

Remnant particles are found in overweight people with high triglycerides. Normalizing triglycerides with weight loss is the recommended treatment to reduce remnant-particle cholesterol elevation and associated risks.

With all this said, triglycerides are important. If you are in need of energy between meals, hormones release triglycerides from your stored fat cells to provide energy for your body. Because triglycerides may be too high for many reasons, it is most important to identify and treat the underlying cause.

If you are overweight, begin a weight reduction plan. If, after reducing your weight your triglycerides are still not in optimum range, medication may be needed. Lowering triglycerides is not something you can do overnight, but losing just ten pounds can help.

Even if you feel fine, having a lipid blood panel done is very important to assess risks and discuss treatments with your physician. High blood pressure and high lipid levels may provide no symptoms until you have a heart attack or stroke.

When Janice was in her late 30's, and after giving birth to three healthy children, a nurse in the office where Janice worked took her blood pressure. This health service was offered to all employees. To her shock, Janice's blood pressure was 280/140. The nurse wanted to take her immediately to a nearby physician. Janice refused. She felt great, brought healthful foods to work for lunch and walked daily for the half hour following lunch. Her father died young of a heart attack, as did his brother. She believed she was healthy and had never considered herself at risk for heart disease. Janice made an appointment for a medical exam and a lipid panel. Her blood pressure remained very high and her cholesterol was markedly elevated at 350! It took a period of 4 months to find the right drugs to stabilize her blood pressure and reduce her cholesterol. Since then, she has regularly taken two blood pressure medications, and a statin to normalize her lipids. Janice had two serious but highly treatable disease processes and no symptoms. Twenty years later, she is healthy, exercising, continuing to eat a low fat healthful diet —and always takes her medications.

Your Heart

♥ Risk modification is done over years; it is a lifetime job. The choices you make every day, many times a day, affect your health. Food choices, exercise, and actually eliminating some foods from your diet entirely will set you in the right direction. Start now by avoiding rich pastries and all fried food. Make healthier meat choices, selecting fish and chicken over red meat. When cooking meat, avoid frying, instead, *boil, broil or bake your meat.* And, exercise daily.

Chapter 5
Female Heart Disease

Women and Heart Disease

Many women do not realize they are at **high risk** for heart disease and early death. Under age 50, heart attacks in women are twice as likely to be fatal as in men. Each year more than 250,000 women die of heart attacks. Six times the number of women die from heart disease than from breast cancer. Many factors weigh into these statistics including hormones.

♥ Research reported in the National Institutes of Health bulletin, *The Heart Truth for Women,* states that by leading a healthy lifestyle, women can lower risks by 82%. You are in charge. This means: regular exercise, healthy weight and not smoking. Also take medications to control other risk factors such as high blood pressure and high cholesterol. What you choose to do and what you eat can improve health and prolong life.

In 2003, the American Heart Association began National Wear Red Day®. With so many women dying each year from heart disease, this movement was formed to bring attention to the problem. Their goal was to educate women and reduce this statistic. For the past ten years, each February, the Go Red for Women events have raised awareness and helped women make strides against heart disease. Fewer women are dying from coronary artery disease now, but it remains the number one threat.

Coronary Microvascular Disease

Early in life, male and female hearts look alike and act the same. With aging, gender differences in disease processes become apparent and contribute to misdiagnosis in women. Men typically develop arterial heart disease that narrows large coronary arteries on the heart surface. Women have the same type of large vessel disease as men, but are also prone to *coronary microvascular disease* — a problem involving the small vessels called arterioles.

Possibly triggered by inflammatory disorders, coronary arterioles in women become stiff and unable to supply adequate oxygen to the heart muscle. Chest discomfort and other symptoms more subtle are often associated with increased activity. Microvascular disease increases your risk for heart attack and sudden death.

A number of health problems cause inflammation including high blood glucose, smoking and chronic infection that also affect men. Additional factors in women are: poorly controlled premenopausal hypertension, anemia and *autoimmune disorders**. All of these problems may contribute to developing coronary microvascular disease. However, the cause of this disease is unknown. The Women's Ischemia Syndrome Evaluation study (the WISE study) provided extensive information for the disorder. Some researchers believe estrogen reduction is a related. Anyone can develop coronary microvascular disease, but inflammatory disorders appear to be a prominent factor and they are more common in women.

Special tests are required to diagnose coronary microvascular disease. Advanced disease may be present, placing the person at risk, yet a *coronary angiogram* — the best diagnostic evaluation for large coronary arteries — can be normal. **If the clinical suspicion for heart disease is high and the angiogram is normal, a "Stress-Echo" is usually recommended to evaluate for microvascular disease.**

Coronary microvascular disease cannot be treated with stents or a bypass, but medications and lifestyle changes are beneficial and life-prolonging. Treatment is similar to that used in large vessel coronary disease:

- Statins to lower cholesterol
- Low dose aspirin to inhibit platelets
- Nitroglycerine to relax and dilate arterioles to improve blood flow and treat chest discomfort
- ACE inhibitors to lower blood pressure
- Beta blockers to lower heart rate and reduce heart stress
- Heart healthy diet, daily exercise, no smoking, weight loss

Note: Autoimmune diseases occur when the body produces harmful antibodies against itself. Examples: Lupus, rheumatoid arthritis, psoriatic arthritis, multiple sclerosis, some thyroid diseases and many others.

Heart Risks in Menopause

Menopause is the biological time when ovary function ceases. Ovaries produce three primary hormones: estrogen, progesterone, and a small amount of the male hormone testosterone. Ovarian production of these hormones stops at menopause precipitating gradual changes in the female body. Not only are there are unrecognized cardiac changes but around age fifty when ovarian function naturally fades, most women begin recognizing additional changes. Some of these are: mood disorder, reduced libido and hot flushes. Without estrogen, bones weaken and silent vascular changes begin and lead to heart disease.

A study at Johns Hopkins examined 2500 women and found those who entered menopause early, before age 46, experienced double the risk of heart attack and stroke. Menopause typically occurs between ages 45-55. Women who smoke enter menopause earlier. Delaying menopause favors a longer healthier life.

When premenopausal women have their ovaries surgically removed, *surgical menopause* symptoms begin abruptly. Starting at a younger age than natural menopause, problems related to estrogen deficiency take a toll on bone health, making osteoporosis more likely. In women lacking estrogen, skin changes become evident with facial wrinkling and vaginal tissue dryness. Head hair may become thinner and facial hair more prominent. In the past, hormone replacement therapy using estrogen, progesterone or a combination of the two was the recommendation. If a *hysterectomy* (surgical removal of the uterus) had been done, estrogen replacement alone could be used. Otherwise hormonal menstrual cycling induced by progesterone was necessary to decrease risk for uterine cancer.

Based on information from the Women's Health Initiative, as of May 2012, the U.S. Preventive Services Task Force recommended no hormone replacement to prevent hot flashes and chronic diseases such as heart disease and osteoporosis. After examining studies over many years, weighing the risks and benefits of taking replacement hormones, the risks were deemed too high to warrant replacement hormones.

Your Heart

Side effects of hormone replacement therapy after menopause:

• Estrogen plus progesterone: increases risks for heart disease, stroke, blood clots, breast cancer, and the risk of dementia doubles.

• Estrogen alone without progesterone: No increased risk for heart disease, but risks increase for stroke and blood clots. Effect on breast cancer is uncertain. Effect on dementia: no protection.

• Most physicians will not order replacement hormones because of the above negative factors.

A study, that may become very important to many women who suffer from menopausal symptoms and osteoporosis, examined breast cancer rates in eleven countries. Because a previous analysis of large long term studies showed a possible correlation to hormone use and increased breast cancer, most women were removed from hormone therapy. As a result, women who might benefit from hormones are not on them. **A new study found no clear link between a reduction in the use of hormone replacement and a decrease in breast cancer.**

Certainly women who have been treated for breast cancer with abnormal cell types with surface markers positive for estrogen and/or progesterone should not take hormone replacements. But with this recent report showing no clear evidence that avoiding hormone replacement reduces breast cancer, a woman's need for hormone therapy can be reconsidered.

If used safely, low dose estrogen therapy could be vital to improving the health of many women. There are increased risks for blood clots, so benefits and risks of taking replacements must be carefully weighed. Still, under specific circumstances hormone replacement therapy may be appropriate. If you have concerns, discuss them with your physician.

A study in Denmark included a thousand women, 500 who took hormone replacement therapy for ten years following menopause and compared health differences with 500 women who took no hormones. Women stopped taking hormones when the Million Women Study showed an association with increased risk of breast cancer. The two groups were evaluated at the end of 10 years and again 6 years later. The endpoints of the study were death or hospitalization for heart attack or heart failure. **Women who took hormone therapy had a significant reduction in mortality, heart attack and heart failure—and no increase in cancer, clots, or stroke.**

Another important Japanese study relates directly to menopausal women, their heart risks, and bone health. This study examined both lipid panels and markers of bone health, including bone density. After menopause, within two years researchers found the total cholesterol went up by 10%, the LDL (bad cholesterol) went up by 20% and the HDL (good cholesterol) went down by 10%. All are negative changes correlated with increasing risk for atherosclerosis.

Within one year, the study group *on hormone replacement therapy showed an improved HDL and a 3% increase in bone density.* Other markers including total cholesterol changed little. Knowing the value of a high HDL and the disabling problems of osteoporosis, doctors may now be willing to reassess the need for hormone replacement therapy in many menopausal women.

Coronary heart disease gradually increases in women after menopause but can also affect younger women who have functional ovaries and continue to menstruate. American Heart Association statistics show heart disease kills 16,000 young women between the ages of 30-55, each year. Women under age 55 may not recognize the symptoms of heart disease. Or, they don't seek medical attention believing they are too young to have a heart attack. Women who have heart attacks are more likely to die from them than men the same age. Since 1995, the rate of heart attacks in women under the age of 60 has risen 25%.

Many variations in coronary artery problems exist. Sometimes there is a congenital narrowing of a single vessel or a weakness in the artery wall. Just like an aneurism in the aorta that splits through some of the layers of the artery (called dissection), the same problem can occur in heart arteries. Of real concern is a report on young women presented at European heart conference this year. Patients from age 16 to 39 without a history of smoking or cocaine use were treated for heart attacks. One was a pregnant woman with a *coronary artery dissection* (the layers of the artery wall split) requiring bypass surgery. Some young women have no disease but experience artery spasms or *vasculitis* (inflammation of the artery) causing pain and ECG signs of ischemia.

These researchers described an upward trend of coronary disease and heart attacks in young women around the world. Many studies have documented under-treatment and delays in care to women presenting with heart attacks. Acute heart attacks in younger women are becoming more common and risk of death is high.

♥ Because heart disease in women is variable, women of all ages including post menopausal women, need to pay attention to symptoms that could indicate heart trouble. **Symptoms some women ignore are: indigestion, dizziness, depression, weakness, jaw aching, sweating, shortness of breath, and of course, chest pain.**

Sudden Death Risks and Causes

After menopause, as estrogen levels drop, women appear to have more risk for heart rhythm abnormalities. It isn't until women become estrogen deficient that they develop atrial fibrillation at the same rate as men.

Women are more likely to develop an electrical variant called *"long-QT syndrome"* than men. The Q-T is a measurement of the electrical impulse recorded on the electrocardiogram (ECG). This variant is known to increase the risk for abnormal beats and sudden death. Rhythm disturbances will be discussed in a later section.

Like men, older post-menopausal women are more likely to develop blockage of the major coronary surface arteries requiring interventions such as *angioplasty* (balloon dilatation) and stents. As stated earlier, women who develop small vessel disease called coronary microvascular disease cannot be treated with stents, because the vessels are too small and medical management is essential. Both large and small types of artery disease may trigger rhythm abnormalities and result in heart attack or sudden death.

Complex gender differences surfaced in a recent study. Researchers at Washington University in St. Louis evaluated 34 human hearts for genetic variation. They saw significant differences in female atria related to 89 genes involved with electrical conduction and heart rhythm abnormalities. Identifying genetic variation in cardiac function and many other disease processes is a prominent area of study with hopes of early identification of problems, prevention and treatment.

The Nurses' Health Study covering three decades and involving more than 100,000 healthy women has provided important women's health information. Recently published information from data collected from the nurse study revealed **women who smoked had a significant rise in the risk for sudden cardiac death.**

Two-thirds of women who die suddenly had no warning. In 80% of cases, autopsy findings show evidence of heart disease. Premenopausal women are less vulnerable to rhythm disturbances under the protection of estrogen.

Additional risks for sudden death:
- Low potassium and magnesium that may result from taking diuretics
- Illicit drug use
- Obesity
- Diabetes
- Drugs may increase abnormal rhythms including some antibiotics

People who die suddenly from heart disease are most likely to die in the early morning hours, between 5-7 a.m. This may be due to genetic variations and body changes related to biological circadian rhythm. Sudden death occurs commonly in both men and women but is more common in those with a history of heart attack in the preceding six months and especially if a large area of the heart was damaged in the first heart attack.

Takotsubo Cardiomyopathy
Another heart problem most often seen in menopausal women under acute stress states is a form of heart dysfunction called *Takotsubo Cardiomyopathy*. This heart problem was first identified in Japan. The name was chosen because the heart shape looks like a takotsubo, an octopus trap.

The actual cause of this disorder is not known but is believed to be related to surges of stress hormones stunning the heart and preventing it from contracting normally. Some call it *stress cardiomyopathy* or *broken heart syndrome*. In animal studies, the presence of estrogen appears to protect the heart, resulting in less cardiac dysfunction under severe stress. This may be why Takotsubo is most often seen in estrogen deficient women between ages 58-75. Younger women lacking estrogen after surgical menopause from ovary removal are also at risk.

The emotional stress of losing a loved one, receiving bad news, or experiencing domestic violence can break your heart—literally. Emotional stress is clearly associated with Takotsubo. The heart weakens in the face of sudden distress and the main pumping chamber of the heart balloons instead of contracting. Symptoms like that of a heart attack occur including chest pain and shortness of breath.

Takotsubo shows electrocardiogram changes that could be mistaken for a heart attack. In addition, there is often a small sharp rise in the blood level of a heart injury marker called *troponin.* In a typical heart attack caused by a blocked coronary artery, the damaged heart muscle cells also leak troponin, but usually in larger amounts.

Based on worrisome symptoms and findings, the cardiologist would likely perform an angiogram which is a fluoroscopic X-ray taken while dye is squirted into the coronary artery. If a blocked artery is found, it would be dilated and stented. It is estimated that in about 10% of women with heart symptoms, the cardiologist finds clear arteries but the ballooning heart of Takotsubo.

Treatment of Takotsubo is similar to other forms of cardiomyopathy. Doctors usually order heart failure medications including beta blockers to reduce heart rate, ACE inhibitors to dilate arteries lowering blood pressure and making it easier for the heart to pump, and diuretics to remove excess fluid. On this drug regimen, most women experience good recovery in two months. Other less fortunate women may be left with reduced heart function and abnormal heart rhythms.

In an 11 year Minnesota study on Takotsubo including 250 women, 20% of them had severe heart failure and low blood pressure. The death rate was higher in women of advanced age with chronic illnesses who developed the cardiomyopathy. At this time, there are no clear guidelines for the best treatment. Research is ongoing.

Stress

♥ **What to do:** Consciously combat stress by learning ways to calm yourself through meditation, Yoga, guided imagery or visualization. Obtain counseling. Make life changes.

Both women and men have significant stress issues. Chronic stress takes a toll on health by reducing immunity, raising inflammatory markers and has also been shown to correlate with hypertension and heart disease. Anxiety, nervous tension, and poor sleep, all add to health problems. Both physical and emotional stress can raise blood pressure.

Mind-body connections are powerful in sickness and in health. No matter where they are, those who practice meditation can enter a state of tranquility, calm their anxieties and experience feelings of physical and emotional well-being. Meditation combined with mental imagery can carry you away from stressful situations and high anxiety, to a place of mental relaxation and peace.

For those unfamiliar with the process of meditation, you learn to focus away from your overload situation. By clearing stress from your consciousness and employing relaxation techniques, you can reduce tension and attain calm inner feelings. Meditation is not considered treatment for hypertension, but it can help—at least temporarily. Most hypertension requires medication to bring readings into normal range, but calming methods can help lower heart rate and blood pressure, relax muscles and provide inner peace.

Traditional Chinese medicine has used many forms of meditation, combining relaxation, movement, breathing and balance techniques. Practiced by large sections of Asian populations, Tai Chi has become popular with all ages in the US and around the world. This graceful martial art form uses slow movements while focusing on deep breathing. Qigong, another ancient Chinese method of health and stress management combines movements, breathing exercises and meditation. Yoga teaches postures, poses, balance, and controlled breathing to enhance flexibility strength and stress reduction. Taking a class is helpful to practice some of these techniques.

One effective form of meditation you can do on your own is guided imagery. With eyes closed, allow yourself to relax completely while forming a mental image of a place or situation you find relaxing. For example: Recalling how you felt at peace with the world while on a seaside vacation. Return there in your mind. Think of the time of day, warmth of the sun, smells, bird songs, beach sand in your toes, the sound of ocean waves. Erase worries from your consciousness. Think of nothing but the peace you have found. Remain there in spirit for a few moments. Try this before bedtime, you may sleep better.

Heart Attacks in Women
When women experience a myocardial infarction, symptoms may be classic with crushing chest pressure, weakness and sweating, or their symptoms may be mild. The following scenario of a patient I cared for will give you a visual image of one lucky woman with an unusual history.

Every person is different. Just because heart pain is usually pressure-like, it doesn't mean sharp pain is not the result of a heart attack. This was very evident in one woman brought in by ambulance screaming in pain. She was 50 years old, thin and dripping wet, having been swimming when her pain began. Swimming laps daily, she appeared physically fit and as though she was experiencing an anxiety attack, not a heart attack.

An immediate electrocardiogram tracing revealed classic findings of a heart attack involving most of the left ventricle. In a rural hospital without a heart specialist, immediate treatment to reduce her symptoms included oxygen, intravenous nitroglycerine, aspirin, morphine and lorazepam to reduce her anxiety. Arrangements were made for a medical helicopter airlift to a hospital more than an hour away. A clot-melting drug was administered intravenously. While waiting for the flight team to arrive, the patient suffered a cardiac arrest from ventricular fibrillation, an oft fatal rhythm. Her heart rhythm normalized after a defibrillator was used to administer an electric shock. A few minutes later, her electrocardiogram normalized and showed no evidence of a heart attack. The clot-melting drug worked! It had opened the coronary artery. When the helicopter lifted off, the patient was stable, comfortable and very much alive.

♥ **What to do:**

From this scenario, you can see why anyone with chest pain should be transported to the hospital by ambulance. Treatment is started en route. If a defibrillator shock is needed to correct an abnormal rhythm, trained medics can do this within seconds while the patient is being transported. If a friend or family member is driving the patient to the ER and a lethal rhythm occurs en route, by the time the patient reaches the emergency center it may be too late.

♥ Women with microvascular dysfunction may have mild or unrecognizable symptoms. Remember, women can have both types of coronary disease. Nagging, recurrent, subtle symptoms must be evaluated. **The symptoms women sometimes recall are: fatigue, poor endurance while walking, lack of energy, chest or abdominal discomfort with activity, jaw pain, and a heavy sensation in the chest.** The symptoms are more likely to occur during exercise and resolve at rest. Don't ignore these symptoms. Coronary microvascular disease may also be seen in men and in diabetics.

Following a heart attack, the risk for having another is very high. The recurrence is high because seldom is coronary heart disease limited to one vessel. Within six years following a heart attack, 21% of men and 33% of women experience a second event. Chances of dying from a second heart attack are high.

To reduce the likelihood of having another myocardial infarction, no tobacco, daily exercise, a healthful low-fat diet and the following medications are recommended:

- Statin to reduce LDL cholesterol to less than 70 mg/dL.
- Daily 81 mg aspirin.
- Beta blocker to reduce the heart workload.
- ACE inhibitor to lower blood pressure and other benefits.
- Based on current information, if you have evidence of heart failure, CoQ10 is a beneficial supplement.

Your Heart

Coronary Artery Disease in Men

Men develop coronary artery disease earlier in life than women. This is because women are somewhat protected against artery changes until about ten years following menopause. Aging and just being male increases risk for coronary artery disease. As in women, the highest male mortality is related to a build-up of cholesterol inside artery walls called atherosclerosis.

Over the past twenty years, there has been a decrease in cardiovascular deaths, probably related to less smoking and better control of blood pressure and cholesterol. However, deaths related to diseased arteries having plaques of fatty material on their inner walls remains the number one killer of both men and women. Each year this cardiovascular disease causes more deaths than HIV and all cancers combined.

Researching the incidence of heart disease in men revealed many sources of disturbing documentation of long-standing and progressive coronary artery disease in young men. Information from autopsies performed on US military causalities during the Korean War revealed 77% of them had visible coronary artery disease, 15% with severe disease. At that time, this silent epidemic was deemed a high public health risk.

Years later, Vietnam War autopsies showed a marked reduction in artery disease findings, 45% vs. 77%. Part of the large difference is thought to be due to the way the disease scoring was performed, there had been an improvement but significant evidence of disease remained.

Heart disease mortality rates peaked in the late 1960's. The incidence has decreased through better understanding of atherosclerosis and reduction of risk factors, but death due to heart disease remains a huge problem. In 1993, in an autopsy study examining atherosclerosis in 111 young male US trauma victims aged 26 +/- 6 years, researchers found 78% had coronary atherosclerosis, with 20% of those having arteries with more than a 50% occlusion; 9% had vessels narrowed by more than 75%. This is very high incidence and high grade of disease in such young men.

To provide accurate comparison, researchers developed standardized descriptions and classifications of coronary disease. These were instituted in an analysis of Armed Forces casualties in recent wars. Overall, researchers found the level of atherosclerosis increased with age and level of obesity. But they found only 8.5% had evidence of coronary disease. The marked reduction is thought to be related to non-standard comparisons in the previous studies of Korean and Vietnam casualties, coupled with improvements due to reduction of risk factors such as stopping smoking.

In the Minnesota Heart Survey tracking trends in heart disease, men were more likely to be smokers and have untreated high blood pressure and high cholesterol. Teenage males, who were inactive, obese and smoked, were at much higher risk for early heart disease than their thin, non-smoking active cohorts.

Low Testosterone

With age, men experience a gradual decrease in testosterone production. Testosterone is an *andro*genic hormone; *andro* means male. This class of hormones contributes to male characteristics such as facial hair, genital development, sperm production, libido and muscle mass. With a drop in testosterone levels, there is an increase in cardiovascular death, just as there is in women after menopause. In one study published in the *Online First Heart Journal*, Professor Kevin Channer, a heart specialist at the Royal Hallamshire Hospital in Sheffield, UK, explained that there are no studies showing normalizing levels of the hormone through supplements are harmful. However, he reported more studies are needed to prove benefit of hormone replacement.

Men with heart failure experience accelerated aging and an *andropause syndrome* due to lack of testosterone production, much like women at menopause who experience a loss of estrogen and menstrual cessation. Some researchers believe testosterone levels decrease with increasing age as part of the natural aging process and should not be treated. Other doctors, and certainly drug companies, say low testosterone levels should be normalized. In the past, many doctors didn't believe *andropause* existed. There is a name for it now, Androgen Deficiency in the Aging Male, (ADAM).

Your Heart

Men with low testosterone blood levels have reduced androgen stimulation. With this, the following symptoms may be present:

- Erectile dysfunction, reduced libido, decreased facial hair
- Psychological symptoms include anxiety, depression, discouragement and irritability
- Muscle and joint complaints, exhaustion, sleep disturbance, weakness, sweating

A recent study reported from the European Society of Cardiology Heart Failure Congress, found one-third of men with systolic heart failure experienced symptoms of androgen deficiency regardless of age, but in men aged 40-59, symptoms were more severe and four times higher than those without heart failure. Additional research in heart failure patients with low testosterone is needed to evaluate use of supplemental testosterone to determine its efficacy in improving quality of life.

To take testosterone, until recently injections were necessary. Now, topical forms can be applied to the skin with ease. High-volume television ads for testosterone replacement for "low-T" have triggered a surge in testosterone prescriptions as a way to enhance virility. Is there a down side?

One study examining testosterone replacement therapy for low testosterone levels had to be stopped because of *increased heart events* in users. Just as some women on hormone replacement therapy experience vascular events such as clots and strokes, there were some detrimental findings in men in the testosterone hormone replacement study. More long-term studies on testosterone replacement therapy are needed to determine lasting effects, both positive and negative.

At this time, testosterone therapy is questionable. Some men want to use more testosterone to improve strength, vitality and virility, even though their hormone levels are normal. By doing so, they may be increasing their risks for coronary artery disease. Another negative side effect of increased testosterone is enhanced growth of prostate cancer cells.

High Risk of Sudden Death

In an interview with *USA Today,* Russell Luepker, professor of public health at the University of Minnesota and spokesman for the American Heart Association, reported autopsy findings in victims of sudden death. The study looked at those less than age 60. Ninety-five percent were men and most of them had heart disease.

In a Minnesota Mayo Clinic study on victims of sudden death, they found coronary arterial disease was much greater in those who died suddenly than in an age/sex-matched control group. In 85% of those dying of sudden cardiac death, the most common finding was a clot occluding an artery (*coronary thrombosis*) over a site of plaque erosion or rupture. Another journal article on sudden death reported about 60% of sudden death is caused by coronary thrombosis, the rest die due to arterial narrowing but without evidence of an occluding blood clot.

Statistics estimate 250,000 people die each year of sudden death and half of them are less than age 65. Many of these deaths can be prevented by early diagnosis, risk reduction and treatment with appropriate medication. Stopping cigarettes is very important.

Erectile Dysfunction Drugs

Many men who have hypertension and diabetes experience erectile dysfunction. Glucose normalization and hypertension control are essential for recovery. But penile erection is a very complex mechanism requiring not only intact circulation and innervation, but the right mental set for arousal.

Under favorable circumstances, erection occurs with the natural release of nitric oxide, a neurotransmitter responsible for increasing arterial blood flow to the penis. At the same time, veins draining the penis contract, trapping the blood and maintaining the erection. If there is a problem with arteries, veins, nerves or brain response, an erection does not occur.

Recent studies contributing to the understanding of maintaining an erection were published in *Proceedings of the National Academy of Sciences.* The study recorded ongoing impulses from physical stimulation and the brain response during cyclic activation of nerves in the penis. Erectile dysfunction drugs act to prolong the neural activation sustaining vasodilatation and erection. Activation of this response by drugs such as Cialis and Viagra lowers blood pressure due to *vasodilatation*. Vessels dilate, become larger, and blood pressure drops. But the blood pressure usually falls less than 10 mmHg and results in no symptoms.

A crisis occurs when nitroglycerine is taken to reduce chest pain after a man has taken an erectile dysfunction drug. Similar to the erectile dysfunction drugs, nitroglycerine is a potent vasodilator. The additive effect of these two medications taken together can lower blood pressure to dangerous levels. Those who use erectile dysfunction medication must be aware of the serious and potentially fatal outcome if nitroglycerine is used for chest pain. **If you are taking a drug for erectile dysfunction and develop chest pain, do not take nitroglycerine. Tell your physician and/or medics about all medications you are taking.**

Hair Loss

A recent report described hair loss in men as a marker for heart disease. The mechanism is unknown. They found those with extensive balding on the top of the head (vertex) had a 48% risk of heart disease as compared to an 18% risk in men who experienced only mild hair loss in the same location. Frontal balding had no association with coronary artery disease.

Seeking Medical Care

Many studies point to higher risks for heart attacks and sudden death in males because men are **less likely to seek medical care, and less likely to treat high blood pressure and abnormal lipids**. Also, men are more likely to smoke cigarettes. If you add obesity, diabetes, unhealthy food choices, stress and excessive alcohol consumption, arteries throughout the body experience accelerated atherosclerosis.

However, men who are thin, active and have normal blood pressure are still at risk for heart disease. The silent vascular narrowing of arteries from lipid abnormalities may not be effectively corrected by food choices and lifestyle. To lower risks, some people require medication to normalize elevated cholesterol levels. A history of family members experiencing early heart attack or sudden death suggests an inherited disorder. This is often familial hyperlipidemia resulting in early vascular narrowing — but there could be other undiagnosed familial problems related to heart structure.

Anabolic Steroid Use

Anabolic-androgenic steroids are a type of drug banned in the sports world. They are *synthetic variants of testosterone.* Prescribed legally for delayed puberty in boys, because of their dangerous side effects, the same products are illegal when used for body building.

Abusers of anabolic steroids usually take them cyclically for months to enhance muscle building. Abuse leads to aggressive behavior, mood swings, anger outbursts and manic behavior. Some reports of paranoid jealousy and rage appear related to the drug. When stopping them, there are reports of both positive mood results, as well depression.

Measurable effects of anabolic steroid drugs are: increased cholesterol levels leading to heart attack and stroke, liver damage, kidney failure, increased risk for prostate and liver cancer, heart enlargement and high blood pressure. In addition: acne, hair loss and reduced sperm count are reported. A commonly abused anabolic steroid purchased on black markets is Dianabol. In the body, this male hormone is metabolized into a form of estrogen causing feminizing changes of breast enlargement and testicle shrinkage.

Your Heart

Anatomy of a Heart Attack

A heart attack happens when one of the following events occurs: plaque or a blood clot fully blocks a coronary artery, or a plaque that has been causing a partial obstruction for years, suddenly breaks open, spilling debris into the blood. The debris is carried downstream and blocks a vessel, preventing blood from reaching a portion of the heart muscle. The heart has no pain receptors, so pain from lack of oxygen is not usually sharp like that of a cut or a burn. Instead, sensation follows blood vessels, radiating into the neck, jaw and inner arms.

Most people describe heart pain as "pressure" or a feeling of having an "elephant sitting on my chest." The discomfort can be sharp, but often, it is dull. Depending on the size of the area of heart damage, a person may have minor symptoms or extreme pressure, feel faint, sweat profusely, feel nauseated, experience shortness of breath or even gasp for air. A heart attack is a *myocardial infarction*. (*Myo* refers to muscle; *cardial* refers to heart; *infarction* refers to tissue death) Once blood flow in a vessel is blocked, oxygen to the muscle downstream is stopped. The area beyond the block will die unless the flow is quickly re-established.

One of the goals of this book is to encourage people to do something before the heart sustains damage. Cell death in the heart is a critical event. The muscle is damaged, pumping action is impaired, and the nerves carrying impulses generating contractions are often injured.

Initially the oxygen-deprived muscle stiffens and does not contract well. When a myocardial infarction damages nerves that are the "electrical wires" of the heart, the result is similar to having a "short" in an electrical circuit in your home. If nerves carrying the paced impulses to trigger the heart beat are damaged, heart block of various kinds may occur. The irritable heart muscle may respond improperly and irregular rhythms occur. Fatal rapid arrhythmias will stop regular contractions. When that happens, blood flow ceases.

Two common lethal rhythms noted in the first section that Dorothy experienced are *ventricular fibrillation* and *ventricular tachycardia*. Both can be reset by a quick electrical

69

shock from a *defibrillator*. Because this treatment must be accomplished quickly and is so effective, small automated defibrillator devices are now being placed in malls, schools and even on airliners. Non-medical personnel are trained to use them. In ambulances, trained medics use defibrillators and can begin other life-saving measures.

Many times patients are in denial. They don't believe it could be a heart problem and don't want to call an ambulance or go to an ER. I have heard many excuses. *It's indigestion. Maybe it's bursitis. I pulled a muscle. It was the burrito I had for lunch. I've had it before and it always went away.* It is better to go to the ER on a false alarm than die. ER and ambulance bills are less costly than a funeral.

Ted didn't smoke or drink, but he thought the four food groups were: steak, French fries, ice cream, and chocolate. At age 62, his eating habits caught up with him. While on a vacation in Florida, one hot, muggy morning, he didn't feel well and thought it was "heat stroke." Back in the air-conditioned motel room, he improved and refused his wife's suggestion to go the hospital. Finally in the middle of that night, he awakened, nauseated and sweating. His wife called 911. Ted stubbornly walked to the ambulance on his own and climbed in, still claiming he was okay. Moments later, the heart monitor went crazy, then flat-lined. The medic started chest compressions. Although Ted couldn't move or see, he heard things going on around him. An assistant called off the time since his heart stopped. One minute...two minutes...He heard one ask, "How far are we from the hospital?"... "Twenty minutes." "Uh-oh, he's not going to make it." After hearing 'five minutes', Ted lost consciousness. CPR continued over twenty minutes. In the ER, he was shocked repeatedly and finally a functional rhythm returned. The cardiologist rushed Ted into the catheterization lab, dilated the artery and placed a stent. Ted almost died (permanently) because he refused to believe he was having a heart attack—until his heart stopped.

If you have a heart attack, the size of the infarction makes a big difference in long-term recovery and function. If the area is small, few or no symptoms occur after recovery. If a large part of the heart is damaged, pump efficiency is lost. Fluid accumulates in the lungs. Oxygen exchange is impaired by the lung congestion and breathing becomes difficult. In other words, you develop heart failure. Extra oxygen helps to relieve respiratory distress. Nitroglycerine absorbed under the tongue or given intravenously relaxes smooth muscle in vessels everywhere and relaxes constricted blood vessels in the heart. Relaxing vessels may allow more blood to flow past the block and reach the ailing heart muscle.

The muscle tissue surrounding the infarcted (dead) area may be stunned due to lack of adequate oxygen. As healing occurs, these injured areas will have some recovery. But the part cut off from all oxygen loses function and heals as scar tissue. The scarred area may become thin and weakens; instead of contracting, it can bulge outward with contractions and reduce the amount of blood pumped out. Heart block causing rhythm abnormalities, and heart failure causing fluid to accumulate in the lungs, may persist after damage by a myocardial infarction. Both heart block and heart failure may also occur through slow progression of heart disease.

The network of arteries in the heart is extensive and somewhat overlapping. Muscle cells near the fully blocked artery can receive some oxygen from nearby arteries but it is often not enough to meet needs. As vessels gradually narrow, sometimes adjacent vessels enlarge and supply some of the area lacking flow. This enhanced arterial flow from nearby vessels is *collateral circulation*.

Following a heart attack, an *echocardiogram* can be done to evaluate the functional ability of the heart. Using sound waves, the cardiac output (the amount of blood pumped out with each contraction), can be estimated. It is usually termed in percentages. For example, a 20% ejection fraction is extremely low, and the person will be severely disabled and life will be shortened. (Note: The normal heart does not empty completely with each beat. A normal ejection fraction is 55-70 %.)

If the person survives a heart attack, changes in the damaged heart muscle and nerves carrying electrical current through the heart can be identified on the electrocardiogram (ECG). About 30% of heart attacks are *silent myocardial infarctions* (not recognized by the person); later when an ECG is performed, abnormalities show evidence of heart injury in the past.

How do I know if I'm having a heart attack?
♥ Memorize these Heart Attack Symptoms:
- A tight squeezing band or pressure around your chest
- Indigestion, nausea and abdominal discomfort
- Discomfort into your neck or down the insides of your arms
- Nausea, perspiration, anxiety, shortness of breath weakness and palpitations
- Discomfort is sometimes perceived as dental or jaw pain, abdominal or upper back pain

♥ What to do
If any of these symptoms occur and last more than a few minutes:
- Call 9-1-1 for ambulance transport to the nearest medical center providing heart care.
- Take an aspirin. The dose recommendations vary, but take at least 160 mg (two baby aspirin). If you have regular adult aspirin on hand, chew and swallow one 350 mg tablet. (Powdered aspirin in packets is now available for quick action in heart emergencies.) Aspirin may save your life. It inhibits the first step in clotting and may help stop the progression of a heart attack.
- If you are already on a blood thinner such as Warfarin or other drugs such as Pradaxa™, ask your physician for recommendations, should you develop chest pain.

Heart attacks can occur at any time, at rest or with vigorous activity. Sometimes a vessel closes with exposure to cold weather, with lifting, climbing stairs or swimming in cold water. You may even be awakened from sleep with chest discomfort.

Knowing many heart attacks occur during early morning hours, medical researchers have recently released information on a remarkable electronic chip that could be of value in many heart patients. The surgically implanted chip can provide very early warnings of impending problems such as critical blood glucose changes or the release of tiny amounts of troponin from damaged heart muscle. The device sends an alert to your smart phone. Many electronic apps are available, even ECG tracings can be sent via your smart phone.

Just because you believe you are physically fit doesn't mean you are not at risk for a heart attack. I have cared for many people who believed they could beat the odds and refused to take a statin drug to lower their "bad" cholesterol levels. Two in particular come to mind, one a distance bicycler halfway through a planned ride across the United States and the other a jogger. They were not hypertensive, overweight or diabetic. As surprising as it may seem, both suffered near-fatal heart attacks.

You can do everything right, eat healthy, exercise, and not smoke or drink, yet develop coronary artery disease. Typically this is because of inherited lipid disorders that require more than lifestyle change to normalize levels. Lifestyle is very important but sometimes it is not enough.

A man who became famous after being an overweight smoker, Jim Fixx, began eating right, quit smoking and advocated exercise in his best-selling 1985 book, *The Complete Book of Running.* Unfortunately, at the age of 52, he died while running. His autopsy showed three major coronary arteries supplying his heart muscle were narrowed by 95%, 85% and 70%. The autopsy also showed extensive arterial damage in his aorta and leg arteries. His pattern was to run ten miles a day. Friends reported he had not complained of symptoms and had not seen a physician in years.

In spite of losing sixty pounds, quitting smoking, running for 17 years, and appearing the picture of health, he suffered a cardiac arrest. Had he taken certain medications, he might have prolonged his life. Jim's father suffered a heart attack at age 35 and died of a second heart attack at age 43. Blood lipid abnormalities run in families. A common disorder is *familial combined hyperlipidemia* resulting in elevations of cholesterol and triglycerides and causes heart attacks at young ages, often before age 50. Statins normalize blood lipid levels, reduce inflammation and reverse artery narrowing. These medications are a proven product of science and may be necessary to reduce your heart disease and stroke risks.

We have many more interventions now than we had 20 years ago, many are life-saving. In the past, fewer medications were available. The beta blocker propranolol revolutionized treatment of angina after its use began in the 1960's. Nitroglycerine, a potent vasodilator, available long before beta blockers, is still used today to interrupt coronary artery vasospasm and reduce chest pain caused by restricted blood flow in the heart. We are fortunate today to have many more effective medications to improve heart function. Sometimes medication is the only treatment when invasive procedures are unlikely to provide improvement.

One of the motivations to share heart information in this book is my own family history. My father had hyperlipidemia. In the late 1950's, following his first heart attack at age 46, the treatment was a week of bed rest in an oxygen tent and blood thinners. In those days, little treatment was available. In the years that followed, he was troubled by angina, intermittent chest discomfort. His physically strenuous job as a railroad mechanic working 12 hour shifts often triggered chest pain. He would become pale, sweaty and have to lie down. After taking nitroglycerine under his tongue, he'd soon feel better and could continue. His symptoms worsened, worry lines marked his face. He required nitroglycerine many times each day. A strong cheerful and creative man, he played the piano and banjo, played with me and my three sisters, told us stories and said, with hard work and determination, we could be anything we wanted to be. We loved watching him paint beautiful oil landscapes. At 52, early one morning he suffered a sudden death while sitting at his easel painting. I was just 18 and found him slumped over and motionless. As he fell forward, a wet streak of paint was dragged across his last picture. — His father, brother and nephew died suddenly. The nephew was only 35 years old.

Today, there is so much more we know, more treatments, interventions before a heart attack occurs. Make choices now to prevent a heart attack. More than 50% of people having heart attacks die before reaching a hospital. If you have chest pain, call 9-1-1. Trained medics save lives en route by providing oxygen to assist breathing, nitroglycerine to dilate the closing vessel, morphine to relieve pain and anxiety, and defibrillation for lethal rhythms. An emergency medic's radio call to the receiving hospital will speed your care upon arrival.

Your Heart

If you decide to have someone drive you, or even worse, you try to drive yourself, the decision is foolhardy. Many people arrive at the ER entrance in cardiac arrest and, even with full resuscitation measures, do not survive.

Learn CPR

♥ Silent heart disease is very common. When a heart attack occurs, the heart muscle cells become damaged from inadequate oxygen. The irritable cells malfunction, disrupting the normal heart beat. Instead of a regular beat, the dying and stunned cells generate abnormal rhythms that do not provide enough pumping action. This results in loss of consciousness and no pulse. Providing temporary pumping action by pushing rhythmically on the chest until medical personnel or defibrillator is available, can save a life. Classes are taught in most communities. Contact your local American Heart Association for more information. Information on the simple Hands-Only ™ CPR method is available online at www.heart.org including video training.

Betty Kuffel, MD

Chapter 8
Diagnosis, Treatments and Healthcare

Health Evaluations
Every heart evaluation begins with a complete history and physical examination. When you visit a physician for a comprehensive evaluation, discuss your concerns about heart disease. You need to be ready with information and questions.

Details of your symptoms, family history, lifestyle, tobacco history, and alcohol use, are all important for a practitioner to assess your symptoms and risks. There are many causes of chest pain and shortness of breath. Because some people are so concerned about what the symptoms might mean, out of fear or anxiety, they do not seek health care. Don't be one of those people. Armed with the information in this book, you will be able to discuss concerns and help your physician do a better job of caring for you.

Heart disease in women can be different and produce a wide array of symptoms that must be carefully sorted out. An annual physical, with or without symptoms, is an important step to take toward living longer.

As we age, our bodies begin to show wear. Joints become arthritic, kidney function may decrease, bladder and prostate symptoms are warning signs, but many treatable illnesses are silent. We know about blood pressure, heart disease and pre-diabetes risks. You may have had these for years without knowing it and all that time your arteries were narrowing and heading you toward vascular health problems. What about thyroid disease? When the gland is failing and the hormone is decreasing, it takes months to years to become symptomatic. During that period changes are evolving, leading to anemia, heart disease and additional problems.

What about breast lumps, cervical cancer, ovarian cancer, other cancers, and osteopenia — if they are diagnosed early you have a chance for focused therapy and longer life. In men, health exams are just as important. Prostate cancer is common and care options can be discussed with a specialist. Blood work can screen for many silent diseases such as high blood glucose, thyroid disease, low vitamin D, and hepatitis C that progresses over twenty years and ends in liver failure.

Your Heart

As part of a medical evaluation, your physician will not only listen to your heart and perform a physical exam but will also order blood work. Starting top to bottom, details related to cardiovascular health may be evident on an exam. As you learned, visible signs such as yellow facial lesions around the eyes often mean lipid problems. Obesity and shortness of breath are obvious to the casual observer, and for a physician, they are red flag alerts to ask about the cardiac risk factors we have discussed.

Obesity precludes some physical exams. For example, abdominal obesity makes it impossible to feel enlargement of the spleen and liver. If abdominal pain is a symptom, imaging may be needed such as an ultrasound or CT scan to define an abnormality.

Electrocardiogram (ECG or EKG)

Basic to each heart evaluation is a recording of the electrical conduction in the heart. This simple test, often called an ECG or EKG, looks at twelve electrical views of the heart. The tracing provides a window into the heart's electrical function. This is a supremely important step in diagnosing heart problems, but it is only one of many tests. A normal ECG does not mean the heart is normal. It only evaluates the electrical system at rest at that moment in time. For a while, even a dying heart may have a normal appearing electrical pattern. The ECG tells us details about the conduction time along the nerve fibers, extra beats, heart rate, and rhythm. Changes are also evident if ventricular or atrial enlargement is present.

Mobile Heart Monitors

To determine if palpitations are dangerous rhythm abnormalities, or if symptoms such as fainting are related to the heart, a battery-operated heart monitor (such as a Holter Monitor) is attached to the patient. The device is worn continuously for 24-48 hours. During this time, the monitor records the electrical activity of every single beat. After the test period, the recording is reviewed for abnormalities. The heart rhythm is then correlated with a diary of activities the patient keeps during the recording time.

If symptoms do not occur during the test period, or if symptoms are infrequent, other devices such as a King of

Hearts Monitor can be used. For up to 30 consecutive days this event monitor can record heart rhythm problems. When symptoms occur, the patient pushes a *record* button and the device saves a recording of the rhythm for the physician to evaluate.

Dynamic Electrocardiogram or Treadmill

This test shows the ability of the heart to function under physical stress. While walking on a revolving belt, electrode-leads attached to the patient's chest are connected to an ECG device recording the heart's electrical activity during exercise. The concept is to stress the heart under controlled circumstances to see how it does — see how the patient does, while being continuously monitored electrically and physically with frequent blood pressure checks.

Hearts damaged by narrowed blood vessels filled with atherosclerotic plaques don't do well. With exercise, the narrowed arteries can't supply enough blood and oxygen to the heart muscle, lungs and working leg muscles. The test will be terminated if any of the following occur: sudden onset of shortness of breath, chest pain, leg weakness or pain, or rhythm abnormalities such as early ventricular contractions, ventricular tachycardia, or if ECG changes show ischemia (inadequate heart blood flow). A failed treadmill usually leads to additional testing.

Echocardiogram

This is a non-invasive ultrasound evaluation of the heart performed by an echo technician or a physician. Heart structures, valves, blood flow, size and even the percentage of blood pumped out with each beat is determined. Thickness of walls, evidence of valve disease and the pericardium (sac around the heart) are evaluated. Sometimes the test is done by a special technique via the esophagus. The *esophageal echocardiogram* procedure uses a probe that is placed within the esophagus, closer to the heart to evaluate delicate structures. This way, the atrial septum can be better visualized to determine if there is a defect remaining from fetal circulation.

Your Heart

Stress Echocardiogram

The *stress echocardiogram* is a procedure performed with a patient walking on a treadmill while the speed and grade are increased at 3 minute intervals. In addition to the monitored treadmill, the patient has a specially trained echocardiogram technician or physician in attendance who performs the heart ultrasound immediately after the patient reaches the maximum point of exercise stress. When the heart reaches a target rate or when severe fatigue occurs (at maximum stress), the patient is assisted to lie down quickly. With the patient lying supine, on their back, an echocardiogram is immediately performed while the heart rate is at its peak.

♥ This test is commonly called a ***Stress Echo***. It is the test of choice for women who present with symptoms suggestive of coronary artery disease. The heart ultrasound is a key diagnostic tool because it can pick up ventricular wall motion abnormalities not seen on other tests. A coronary angiogram and electrocardiogram may appear normal in a person with *coronary microvascular disease*. The Stress Echo will show abnormal heart wall motion.

This test is effective in evaluating disease in the larger coronary arteries, but is essential in the diagnosis of microvascular disease often missed by other tests.

Nuclear Stress Test

When imaging is important to make a diagnosis, or to evaluate function and blood flow in the heart, a special test using a radioactive dye (Thallium or sestamibi/Cardiolite) can be used. This test involves evaluating the heart at maximal exercise and again at rest.

The heart rate is raised by having the patient walk on a treadmill, pedal a stationary bike, or by injecting a medication to stimulate the heart rate. When the patient reaches their maximal heart rate from exercise or medication, the radioactive-tagged dye is injected into a vein and carried throughout circulation to enhance visibility of the working heart. A special imaging machine detects and records the radioactive substance within the heart muscle. Areas of the heart not receiving adequate blood flow are seen on the heart images. The size of the heart and its pumping ability are also documented, including the ejection fraction, showing the ventricular output.

Later, after the patient is fully rested, another dose of the radioactive dye is injected and the heart is scanned again. Exercise-images are compared with rest-images to assess for evidence of inadequate blood flow during exercise indicating arterial blockage.

Computed Tomography Angiogram
Computed tomography angiography is also called a *CT angiogram*. This low-risk, non-invasive CT X-ray scan is evolving as a major adjunct in evaluating people with chest pain. Using an intravenous dye to provide images of the inside of coronary arteries, the study is even being used by some metropolitan emergency rooms to evaluate patients who arrive with chest pain. The study is a shift away from invasive cath-lab angiography. In some patients with chest pain, information from the CT angiogram can eliminate the need for hospitalization and avoid the invasive heart catheter procedures. Computed tomography angiography has been available for years in some major facilities but low availability limits its broad use.

Heart Cath/Coronary Angiogram
The combination of symptoms and an electrocardiogram often trigger this study. It requires an invasive cardiologist and a team of specially trained support staff. This procedure is the gold standard diagnostic procedure used to evaluate chest pain. A heart cath is only available in larger hospitals and heart centers. If warranted and close enough to intervene, the patient may be rapidly transferred to a hospital offering the service. Importantly, this procedure provides both diagnosis and intervention capabilities with the ability to open a closed vessel and prop it open with a stent.

If someone goes to a physician or an emergency room and is found to be having a heart attack, rapid intervention is needed to clear the blockage and restore blood flow to the heart muscle. Each passing minute means more heart damage is occurring. Speed Counts — *Time is Muscle*.

While preparing the cath-lab where the procedure is done, medical treatment is started. Interventions include: intravenous access, nitroglycerin to relax and dilate the heart arteries, aspirin or other clot inhibitors, oxygen and blood tests that measures troponin.

If there is a delay, such as a long distance to a heart hospital or a waiting time because the cath lab is in use, then *thrombolytic* therapy is warranted. To understand the word, look at the two components: *thrombo* means blood clot; *lytic* means lysis or melt. The medication melts the clot and opens the vessel, re-establishing blood flow to the heart muscle until an additional intervention is accomplished. Melting the clot may clear the blockage and save heart muscle, just as it saves brain tissue when effective in clearing the clot causing a stroke.

When the angiogram and angioplasty dilatation procedures are done by the heart specialist, the area where the catheter is inserted is anesthetized, much like a dentist numbs the area around a tooth for a dental procedure. Then the artery is punctured and a catheter is threaded via the artery to the heart. The access may be through the femoral artery in the groin, or the radial artery in the arm. This long flexible catheter is about the diameter of spaghetti. Under the fluoroscopic guidance of real time X-ray, the cardiologist advances the catheter while watching its movement as it curves over the arch of the aorta to the location where the large artery exits the left ventricle.

Here, just outside the aortic valve, openings into each coronary artery are identified and entered. Squirts of dye visible on X-ray fill the arteries as the heart is beating. The interior of the arteries is shown by following the track of the dye. Any narrowing inside the arteries is visible and measurable.

Angioplasty and Stents: Opening a Blocked Artery

In a balloon angioplasty and stent procedure, under fluoroscopic X-ray visualization, the cardiologist passes a thin catheter into the tightly narrowed or blocked artery. The unique catheter is designed with a tiny flat balloon around the outside near the tip. When the cardiologist has it in position, the balloon is inflated and stretches open the blocked area. Once blood flow is re-established, stents that look like tiny springs are placed within the exact blockage location propping the artery open. Sometimes, more than one high-grade narrowing is seen and multiple stent procedures must be done.

The stents remain in place forever. Following this procedure, medications to reduce the risk of blood clots and stent closure are required for long periods. Aggressive lowering of lipids and other measures such as exercise and healthy food choices are essential to keep the stents from closing.

Not all coronary arteries can be dilated and stented. Some are technically impossible to enter or open. In some cases there are so many diseased vessels, the patient is referred to a heart surgeon for a vascular bypass procedure of many vessels.

Coronary Artery Bypass Graft Surgery
As the name indicates, the diseased portion of the artery is bypassed. This is accomplished using a vein or artery from another area of the body. The replacement vein or artery is stitched in place to bypass the diseased portion of the coronary artery. First, the narrowed area of the coronary artery is identified. Then, one end of the graft vessel is stitched above the blockage and the other end below, bypassing the blocked area. Blood flows through the newly attached tube to reach the area lacking adequate flow. The new graft is evaluated to assure enough blood flow has been established. Another name for the procedure is *revascularization.*

If a vein graft is used, the vein typically is taken from a leg. If a small artery graft is used, typically it is an arm artery or preferably the internal mammary artery in the chest. If the internal mammary artery is used, it is not cut free; instead the distal part is stitched in below the blockage. Results with this procedure are excellent.

Since the advent of the stent procedure, fewer coronary artery bypass grafts are being done. However, stents do not replace the procedure. Coronary bypass grafts are still the treatment of choice in adults with multi-vessel coronary artery disease as is often the case in diabetics and smokers.

In the hands of highly trained heart surgeons, the coronary artery bypass procedure has saved many lives. It is one of the most commonly performed operations in the world. The hope would be that one day we will have little need for a bypass because of the healthy choices the population chooses beginning in childhood.

In the past, coronary bypass procedures required a "heart-lung machine" to pump oxygenated blood around the body and brain while surgeons worked on the un-beating heart. This procedure is called *cardiopulmonary bypass*. When the surgical procedure is completed, the heart is restarted, the cardiopulmonary bypass is discontinued, and the chest is closed. The heart-lung-machine is needed for many heart surgeries such as valve replacements, some coronary bypass grafting, heart transplants, and congenital heart defect repairs.

Recently, whenever possible, coronary bypass grafts were done "off-pump." This means the surgeon placed the tiny sutures around the artery grafts with the heart still beating. Motion of the beating heart makes the procedure technically difficult for the surgeon but has advantages for the patient.

In a Cleveland Clinic study using off-pump coronary bypass grafting there was a marked reduction in post-operative brain dysfunction called *vascular dementia*. This was coupled with similar outcomes related to mortality and stroke when compared with coronary bypass grafts done using the cardiopulmonary bypass machine.

Note: *Vascular dementia* has many causes. After Alzheimer's, decreased blood flow resulting in brain injury is the most common cause of dementia. A 2013 study reported at the American College of Cardiology from the University of Prague, researchers looked at on-pump vs. off-pump outcomes including: stroke, heart attack and kidney failure. Even in the highest risk patients with additional health problems, *best results were noted in the off-pump group* with half of the negative outcomes.

Anytime a procedure is done on the heart, it is critical and life-threatening, even though life-saving is its goal. Every precaution is taken to maintain blood flow to vital organs and avoid brain damage due to low oxygen delivery. Because memory impairment can occur after these procedures, much research has been done to reduce the complication. In a National Institutes of Health report by V. R. Challa, as high as 38% of patients had memory loss after a bypass procedure. The cognitive decline may be related to toxic neural changes from micro-fat-emboli to the brain occurring silently during the surgery.

Prior to cardiac surgery it is customary to evaluate the carotid arteries in the neck. Sometimes occlusions in the carotid arteries must be corrected before heart surgery can be done in an attempt to decrease the risk of intra-operative stroke.

The bottom line is this: Advanced heart disease is a life-threatening problem with risks impacting the entire the body. With coronary artery disease, you have a similar risk for developing the same process in all the arteries of your body. This includes those in the legs, aorta, kidneys, carotids and brain. Doing any kind of surgery on someone with wide-spread artery disease carries high risks which must be discussed with the patient and addressed by the heart and anesthesiology teams.

♥ Visiting Your Physician
Personal Health History
At your first visit with a physician it is customary to provide a complete health history. Be prepared to provide the following information:

- Family history of inherited or familial disorders such as early heart disease, sudden death, cancer, depression and other mental health disorders, diabetes, strokes, alcoholism and cancer.
- Tell your physician the cause of death of family members. It may relate to your health.
- A list of all your surgeries and the dates.
- A medication list with dosages, including supplements, health food and over-the-counter products. Bring your bottles with you.
- Report history of smoking and other tobacco use. If you use tobacco, request assistance to help you quit.
- A list of immunizations: Request immunizations, especially for tetanus, pertussis (whooping cough) and influenza.
- Discuss other immunizations as appropriate for age. Example: pneumococcal (pneumonia) and shingles.

- General health evaluations: mammograms, pap smears, colonoscopy, bone density evaluation.
- Report other concerns appropriate to age such as: contraception, vaginal dryness, hair loss.
- Report domestic abuse and history of child abuse–both contribute to health risks.
- Be prepared to discuss your heart disease risk factors including how much alcohol you drink.
- Discuss skin screening exam for abnormalities such as melanoma and other skin cancers.
- Travel history is important for some disease processes, even heart disease. (Ex. Chagas disease is a parasitic illness that can cause heart damage. It is spread by insect bites in South America and southern Texas.)

♥ **Obtain a copy of your ECG, health history and drug list**. Carry them with you when you travel. Dentists and other healthcare professionals need your health history and med list.

♥ **Recommended annual laboratory tests to identify many silent diseases:**
- Fasting Lipid Panel — Provides levels of Total Cholesterol, LDL, HDL, Triglycerides and calculates your risk ratio.
- Comprehensive Metabolic Panel —— Evaluates: glucose, liver function, kidney function, electrolytes such as sodium, potassium and calcium.
- Vitamin D level.
- Complete Blood Count (CBC) — Evaluates: white blood cells, red blood cells, platelets; evaluates immune status and checks for anemia.
- Thyroid Panel, including Thyroid Stimulating Hormone (TSH) — Evaluates for both underactive and overactive thyroid.
- Hemoglobin A1c — Evaluates glucose control over the preceding three months; used in diagnosis and management of diabetes.
- Other: Men discuss Prostate Specific Antigen (PSA), a prostate blood test that rises in prostate cancer; testosterone level if symptomatic.

Silent diseases include many disorders. Some of them are: high cholesterol, high triglycerides, low HDL, high blood glucose, kidney failure, low vitamin D, many types of anemia and blood disorders including clotting abnormalities, high or low thyroid, and prostate cancer.

Before you consult a physician, prepare a list of questions and notes so you do not forget to discuss symptoms or concerns.

Your Heart

Chapter 9
THE ARTERIES

Carotid Disease and Stroke

While the primary focus of this book is coronary artery disease, the same guidelines apply for prevention, treatment and reversal of artery narrowing from atherosclerosis no matter where the disease occurs. People with heart disease are very likely to have related problems elsewhere in their bodies. This section can help explain associated problems and why it is important to seek appropriate medical care.

Because strokes are the leading cause of adult disability in the US and the fourth leading cause of death, it is also important to address choices that can lower stroke risks.

Carotid arteries arise from the aortic arch soon after the large artery leaves the heart and just before it curves downward to the supply the rest of the body. The carotid arteries provide blood to the head, neck and brain. When the large important carotid vessels develop disease, they become narrow, irregular inside and may close entirely. As this happens slowly over years, an amazing circle of vessels at the base of the brain can shunt blood around to the side of the brain no longer supplied by the blocked vessel, thus avoiding a large stroke.

Unfortunately, in most cases strokes occur suddenly when bits of cholesterol or clots let go from a diseased carotid vessel and enter the blood stream. This debris is carried into arteries supplying the brain. In an instant, particles can block an artery and immediately stop blood flow. Similar to a *heart attack*, this *brain attack* is called a stroke and results in loss of neurologic function.

Neurologic function is fascinating and complex. Stroke symptoms vary immensely from difficulty swallowing and subtle clumsiness, to loss of balance and complete inability to walk or speak.

If a blocked brain vessel is small and only supplies a small portion of the brain, minor neurologic deficits occur, such as hand weakness on one side of the body. However, if a large area of the brain is affected, especially if the part of the brain controlling breathing is impaired, the person suddenly loses consciousness and dies.

Sometimes a *transient ischemic attack* develops instead of a stroke. People who know about this problem call the episodes TIAs because it is much easier to say. The problem occurs when blood flow to a portion of the brain temporarily stops. Symptoms may include a sudden facial paralysis, a vision change, trouble speaking, confusion or problem walking. Unlike strokes that result in permanent disability, the symptoms of a transient ischemic attack are just that, transient. They dissipate leaving no residual damage.

A transient ischemic attack is a warning. It means you are more likely to have a stroke in the future than someone who has not experienced the temporary problem. You need to see a doctor for a full evaluation. If the source of the clot is identified, an intervention may be done to prevent a stroke resulting in permanent disability.

If you experience any of the symptoms mentioned, call 9-1-1 immediately or see your doctor even if the symptoms quickly resolve.

A person having an embolic stroke caused by floating clots or cholesterol pieces, may experience the same symptoms as those associated with this type the transient attack. But instead of resolving, the neurologic impairment persists. Evidence of the brain injury is visible on CT and MRI scans. With luck after a stroke, over time partial function and mobility are recovered. Typically, there is residual damage. Some strokes are small with few symptoms. Other times they are devastating with marked loss of function, mobility and mental capabilities.

Note: Headaches are not common symptoms of either transient attacks or strokes caused by blockage. **If you develop an unusual sudden headache, you need to seek medical attention immediately.** Middle-aged women are of prime age for a different type of stroke caused by a weakened vessel that ruptures and bleeds into the brain, called a *hemorrhagic stroke*.

Migraines are a specific type of headache resulting from reactive brain vessels accompanied by intense pain, and associated with nausea, vomiting, sensitivity to light and sound. A worrisome headache called a *complex migraine,* results in temporary paralysis. People with migraine headaches of this type should have a full evaluation by a neurologist.

♥ What to do
The National Stroke Association recommends **F.A.S.T.** as an easy way to recall what to look for and do if someone is having a stroke:

F=Face – Ask the person to smile. Is one side of the face drooping due to paralysis?

A=Arms – Is the person able to raise both arms and hold them up?

S=Speech – Is the person able to repeat a sentence after you, without slurred or garbled speech?

T=Time – Don't waste time. Call 9-1-1.

Always call 9-1-1 if you experience stroke symptoms. Just as in heart attacks, immediate treatment is the key to limiting damage. If there is no delay in arriving at an Emergency Room, many strokes can be treated with clot melting drugs to restore function.

Surgery called a *carotid endarterectomy* may be necessary to clear an irregular area or narrowing in a carotid artery. *Endo* pertains to inside, *arter*=artery, *ectomy*=removal. This procedure clears atherosclerotic plaques from the inside of the vessel. The surgery reduces the risk for stroke and could be life-saving. Sometimes this procedure must be performed prior to other major surgical procedures to decrease the risk of a stroke occurring during the planned surgery.

Cerebrovascular Accident is the most commonly used term for a stroke. It is generic and does not tell you what kind of stroke occurred. The word, *cerebrovascular,* identifies the location and type of problem. *Cerebro*=brain, *vascular* pertains to blood vessels. In this case, the term doesn't tell you if it is an arterial or venous stroke. But strokes are typically caused by blocked arteries.

Other related terms and causes:

Cerebrovascular disease: caused by blood vessel narrowing; a cause of memory loss.

Cerebral Infarction: areas of brain cell death due to blocked blood flow.

Ischemic stroke: brain injury due to lack of oxygen.

Hemorrhagic stroke: caused by a ruptured blood vessel and bleeding into the brain.

Embolic stroke: caused by debris which floats in the blood and blocks a brain artery.

Thrombotic stroke: caused by a blood clot *(a thrombus)* in a brain artery.

Stroke symptoms typically occur without warning unless preceded by a transient ischemic attack resulting from the same vascular location. The area of the brain lacking oxygen dictates the resulting symptoms.

Left Brain Stroke

A clot or cholesterol particle from a diseased left carotid artery is carried into the left brain. Blockage in a *left brain artery* may result in:

- Weakness or paralysis on the *right side* of the body: right face, right arm and/or right leg.
- Loss of speech: Speech in most right-handed people is located in the left brain, so in left brain strokes there is usually an inability to formulate words and express thoughts.

Right Brain Stroke

Blockage in a *right brain artery* may result in:

- Weakness or paralysis on left side of the body.
- Cognitive deficit (inability to solve problems).
- Left-sided "neglect" is when the person fails to see objects on the left and may fail to eat food located on left side of plate.
- Serious safety problems and falls occur because of memory loss.
- Impulsive behavior, mood changes and speech problems are common.

Speech and language centers in the brain are complex. There are at least five interactive areas, so problems speaking and understanding can occur with either left or right brain strokes. Lack of swallowing may occur with strokes on either side and is a serious problem.

Your Heart

Preventing a stroke is critical to long-term health and sometimes life itself. If oxygen is blocked even for a few minutes, brain cells die and permanent damage results.

♥ Just as you would with heart attack symptoms, anyone with stroke symptoms should see a doctor immediately. Call 9-1-1. Don't wait. The sooner you get to an Emergency Center that can treat you, the better. Many facilities have stroke procedures in place including immediate neurology consult via the Internet or telemedicine. If you reach medical care soon enough, you may be a candidate to receive a clot melting drug formulated to clear all the devastating effects.

Blanche fell asleep feeling well and without symptoms, but upon awakening, she was unable to speak or move her right arm and leg. Sometime during sleep, she experienced a left brain stroke leaving her with paralysis and inability to communicate. Unable to call for help, she fell to the floor when trying to get out of bed. A family member found her. Medics reported she was minimally responsive with a blood pressure of 230/120. The last time she was seen normal was at midnight, 8 hours earlier.

In this situation, time of the stroke event is unknown. Time eligibility for the clot melting drug Alteplase is within 3-4.5 hours of the stroke. If the time is unknown or is documented to be greater than the stroke guideline time, no drug is given. This sounds harsh if there is some hope of improvement. However, extensive studies have shown the best benefit is in people under the age of 80 and within 3-4.5 hours of symptom onset. There are significant bleeding risks with clot- melting drugs, including brain bleeds. Not everyone is a candidate for this treatment.

The American Heart Association and the American Stroke Association released updated stroke guidelines in January 2013. Since 2007, when clot melting treatment was started, a number of updates have occurred. Current guidelines include:
- Transport patient to properly prepared hospital.
- Perform stroke evaluation scale to determine measurable physical findings.

- Vital sign requirements: a blood pressure below 185/ 110.
- Immediate studies include brain scan and blood tests.
- All examinations in the ER to take less than an hour.
- No contraindication that might result in a bleeding crisis (example: recent surgery).
- Time less than 4.5 hours since the stroke and tPA is administered intravenous within an hour.

In the right setting and technical availability, a clot melting drug may be given directly into the affected artery. This limits exposure to the rest of the body but requires a highly skilled invasive radiologist to perform the procedure. If given intravenously, the clot buster is carried throughout the body increasing risks for bleeding, so in many circumstances, the drug may not appropriate.

Stroke patients need complete neurological and medical evaluations to fully determine their stroke deficit before beginning rehabilitation. Physical and speech therapy and swallowing evaluations may be needed. Very important, too, is the search for a cause so interventions can begin to ward off worse disability and future strokes. Some tests are: an electrocardiogram to look for rhythm abnormalities, ultrasound scan of carotid arteries to look for irregularity and narrowing, and heart ultrasound (echo) to look for diseased heart valves and clots inside the heart that might have caused the stroke.

Stroke survivors who smoke are at great risk for not only another stroke but at higher risk for heart attack and death than those who have never smoked. An American Heart Association report in the journal *Stroke* indicated current smokers had a 42% higher risk for poor outcomes. So, quitting at anytime begins risk reduction.

Physical disability after strokes may be mild or result in such severe damage the person is unable to provide self care. There is hope for recovery but progress and improvement are variable.

In a recent study using hyperbaric oxygen for stroke patients, even years after the stroke occurred, increased oxygen delivered to the brain resulted in major functional improvements. In addition to being used for stroke care, high pressure oxygen chambers may provide some benefit in patients with traumatic brain injuries. The most common application for hyperbaric oxygen is to use high pressure oxygen to saturate tissues of those experiencing deep diving related injury and low oxygen distribution, such as in carbon monoxide poisoning. Research is ongoing for brain treatments. Use is limited to regional centers where hyperbaric chambers are located.

With little awareness the problem exists, some people have many small strokes over time causing minimal functional loss. If the strokes are not stopped by identifying and treating the source, and controlling high blood pressure, a disorder called *multi-infarct dementia* occurs. The person loses more and more cognitive function until memory is severely impaired. Some may be ambulatory but have such severe memory loss they require 24/7 care.

Congenital Heart Defect and Stroke
There are many birth defects involving heart and blood vessels. These problems result from abnormalities in development, chromosomal syndromes and genetic mutations. A common disorder is present at birth but not diagnosed until the individual has a stroke. The problem is related to aberrations in fetal circulation that fail to attain adult circulation once the infant begins breathing and is no longer receiving blood from the placenta.

Fetal circulation overview
In the uterus, the lungs do not supply the fetus with oxygen. Instead, maternal circulation via the placenta carries oxygenated and nutrient-rich blood to the developing child through the umbilical cord *vein*. Like the pulmonary veins in adult circulation, the fetal umbilical vein carries oxygen–rich blood. Two umbilical arteries carry blood back to the placenta. Circulation of fetal blood passes *from the right atrium directly into the left atrium* (through the *foramen ovale*) thus bypassing the non-breathing fetal lungs.

Immediately after separation from the mother and after the baby takes a few breaths, pressure changes within the child's cardiopulmonary system occur. Like in adult circulation, the baby's left atrium fills with blood returning from now-breathing lungs, and closes the special fetal door, the *foramen ovale*, between the atria. This ends one part of fetal circulation as blood is oxygenated by the newborn's lungs.

Patent Foramen Ovale
There are times when the hole in the atrial septum doesn't properly close. When this happens, the hole is called a *patent foramen ovale (PFO)*. *Patent* means open. Many people go through life not knowing their foramen ovale did not close at birth. Some studies show that one third of all adults have PFOs without symptoms. A serious problem arises when the opening between the atria persists and for some reason a venous clot forms and travels in the blood stream to the heart.

The lungs act as a filter. If a clot lodges in the lung it is called a *pulmonary embolus*. With a hole between the atrial chambers, the floating venous clot may go through the PFO from the right atrium directly into the left atrium and enter arterial circulation bypassing the lungs. The PFO is usually small and only when pressure is increased inside the chest such as with a cough or straining with a bowel movement does the clot spurt through from right to left in to the arterial circulation. Pumped out of the left ventricle, the clot can travel to the brain or other organs, resulting in a stroke or infarction wherever it occludes an artery.

Note: The PFO is one of many possible congenital atrial septal malformations. Larger holes that occur when the septum doesn't form properly—*atrial septal defects,* may be associated with strokes, too. But, additional serious problems related to lung pressures and mixing of oxygenated and de-oxygenated blood also occur and may not be diagnosed until adult age like PFOs.

While evaluating a patient in his office, a physician suddenly became unable to speak. His staff brought him directly to the emergency department. There, following stroke protocol, a neurologist immediately evaluated him and instituted treatment. The physician met protocol guidelines and was deemed a candidate for the clot melting drug tPA. Within 2 hours of completing the drug, his speech returned and eventually all evidence of his neurologic deficit cleared. A previously undiagnosed PFO was identified and a closure procedure performed. Being treated immediately with the clot melting drug was the key to his successful outcome and return to his medical practice.

A PFO is diagnosed with a special heart ultrasound study: either an echo with a bubble study or an *esophageal echo.* The communication between the atria is evident with either study. In the bubble study, bubbles are visible crossing through the hole. With the esophageal ultrasound, the hole can be identified via a small probe inserted inside the esophagus in close proximity to the heart. In the skilled hands of an invasive cardiologist, closure can be done by deploying a button-like device via a vessel to seal the hole and stop further stroke symptoms.

Aortic Disease
The largest artery in the body is affected by the same disease process as the much smaller coronary or leg arteries. Disease throughout this vessel causes weaknesses in the wall. Bulging and tearing of the layers of the aorta increases the risk for rupture. An abdominal ultrasound should be done in older people and those known to have peripheral artery disease to evaluate for a weakness or bulge resulting in an *aneurism.* A rupture is usually fatal. If diagnosed before a rupture, treatment involves the surgical insertion of a large stent or replacement with a graft. Inherited disorders unrelated to atherosclerosis can cause vascular disease with vessel wall weakness and aneurisms.

Peripheral Artery Disease
Coronary arteries and arteries throughout the body develop atherosclerosis with stiffening and narrowing. When this occurs in the largest artery — the aorta — narrowing can extend all the way to the leg arteries. With reduced blood flow to leg muscles, leg pain occurs from lack of oxygen, much like heart pain occurs from partially blocked coronary arteries.

Weakness, pain in the calf, and lack of walking endurance are symptoms of peripheral artery disease brought on by inadequate blood flow. When circulation is inadequate, foot and leg pain can be severe. The limb becomes hairless, toe nails thicken and muscles atrophy. When sitting with knees

95

bent and feet hanging down, the leg turns a dark reddish color and may feel numb. Toes may feel cold and turn purplish. If arteries become blocked, the limb dies. The effect of no circulation is gangrene, dead tissue and amputation is required.

Just as coronary arteries can be opened by balloon angioplasty and stents, these distal leg arteries can be treated by similar methods. They can also be bypassed or replaced with grafts using small tubes woven from a special fabric that resembles the flexible hose used to carry hot air from a clothes drier to the outside. Even the aorta can be replaced with a similar fabric graft.

Following invasive procedures to clear or bypass leg arteries, it is essential the patient not smoke and not use tobacco of any kind. This is true for heart procedures, too. A statin prescription that is followed carefully, along with daily aspirin, result in a lower incidence of graft or stent closures. This means fewer amputations. Keeping the artery open is the goal. To do this the risk load must be reduced. The patient must stop smoking and all tobacco use along with being placed on a regimen to stop progression and reverse arterial narrowing. Smoking sabotages stent and bypass procedures.

Prevention is the key. Diabetics are prone to vascular disease with reduced blood flow to the extremities inhibiting healing and increasing risk for amputation. Although interventions and bypasses can provide relief, problems continue. Severe peripheral artery disease is most often seen in smokers. If the patient continues to smoke, their outcomes are worse than non-smokers.

Many different approaches and medications to improve leg circulation are used. Blood thinners reduce clotting risks and help keep the diseased vessels open. Doctors may prescribe aspirin or other platelet-blocking medications to decrease clotting. Statins help by reducing progression and in some cases help reverse the disease. Trental (pentoxifylline) is a unique drug that alters RBCs, making them more flexible and able to squeeze through narrowed vessels thus carrying needed oxygen to tissues. Pletal (cilostazol) helps to improve blood flow.

We have discussed the various locations of arterial narrowing as if they are separate diseases but they are a continuum of the same disease. Someone who has heart disease, carotid disease or peripheral artery disease, has risks for arterial narrowing throughout their body. This is usually the cause of kidney failure, too.

Cardiovascular disease affects nearly 40% of Americans.
With aging, there are changes in all arteries. However, octogenarians with a history of healthy eating and active lifestyle have strong hearts and excellent circulation. We can't choose our parents, but we can make choices that improve our longevity.

♥ <u>You will be healthier from head to toe if you</u> —
- Exercise every day
- Normalize blood pressure
- Do not use tobacco
- Attain normal cholesterol and blood sugar levels
- Eat healthy
- Maintain a normal weight
- Lower your stress

Betty Kuffel, MD

Chapter 10
Keys to Living Longer

Longevity and Exercise

After reading about all the risks associated with cardiovascular disease, you'll probably agree there are things you can begin doing now to increase your chances of living a healthier, longer life. A recently published medical study noted how advanced planning can change the course of your life. Americans are living longer, but not always better. If born today, current life expectancy is seventy-eight, but with longer life more people are dealing with chronic diseases. The goal should be to begin modifying your risks as soon as possible so you not only live longer but are healthier. Developing fitness in middle-age, even if exercise has never been a priority for you, can help reshape your personal health landscape and make later years more vibrant.

In a long term study of 18,000 people beginning in 1970, most who were the *least fit* at the time of their middle-aged checkup had developed some of the following conditions early in the aging process: dementia, diabetes, heart disease, and colon or lung cancer. Those who were *most fit* in their forties and fifties typically did not develop chronic illnesses *until the final five years of their lives,* instead of 10 to 20 years earlier like the less physically fit individuals.

By looking at the big picture of life, we know exercise is beneficial in not only delaying illness but also in adding years of enjoyment to your life. Even walking half an hour a day can improve your overall mental and physical health. Longevity without dementia is determined by mental and social involvement in combination of genetics and fitness.

An article reviewing 45 studies published in the *Journal of the National Cancer Institute* in 2013, examining physical activity in people with cancer, emphasized the benefits of exercise. In exercisers, there was a decrease in *all-cause* mortality, including cancer-related deaths. Many of the studies involved women with breast cancer. With exercise, insulin levels improved, inflammation decreased and cells known to attack tumors increased — all very positive outcomes resulting from exercise.

Muscles strengthen with exercise. Balance improves. But another important benefit is improved blood flow to organs including the brain. Studies even show fit animals not only experienced improved memory; they generated new neurons in areas of the brain involved with learning.

We all have excuses for not finding time to exercise. However, if you evaluate your interests and abilities, there is probably some exercise you can do to remain active, even if you have physical problems that interfere. Consider these:

- Water exercises for individuals with joint and balance problems can increase muscle strength and also be relaxing.
- If you have joint or back problems, consider a non-weight bearing exercise such as riding a stationary bicycle.
- Talk with your physician for more suggestions.
- Maybe a consultation with a physical therapist or fitness trainer could set you on a course to improve muscle conditioning, balance, and overall health.

Cognitive skills and creativity improve with a wilderness experience and increased exercise. A study on hikers documented significant problem-solving benefits when they were tested after spending four days in a rural environment disconnected from all their electronic devices. Enrolled in a nature immersion outing and separated from televisions, smart phones and the Internet, they experienced lowered stress, lowered blood pressure and improved brain function. Plan a nature adventure soon and try to make exercise a part of your everyday life.

If you say, *"I'm too tired to exercise"* — recent studies have found that exercise energizes people, even those undergoing cancer treatments. Remember, exercise doesn't have to be vigorous. Even a slow walk outdoors in the sunshine will brighten your outlook on life, increase bone-density to ward off osteoporosis, strengthen muscles, improve balance and help you live a longer healthier life.

Betty Kuffel, MD

The World Health Organization recommends 3-5 hours of endurance training per week to prevent chronic disease and improve overall health. Before starting any exercise program, it is smart to consult your health practitioner. To begin with, try a walking program. As your endurance increases, add distance and speed. There are many alternatives if you have joint problems.

Consult your doctor before beginning any advanced cardio-fitness regimen, especially if you are new to exercising. Strenuous cardiac fitness requires bursts of vigorous activity to raise your heart rate and improve endurance.

If you are short on time, but want to stay fit, consider the SIT and HIT workout recently published in *The Journal of Physiology*. It is rigorous but shows how cardiovascular conditioning can be achieved in less than one-third the time required by most programs. Using a simple stationary bicycle or spinning cycle, you can accomplish a lot of conditioning in a shorter time by following the study Sit or Hit format. (Note: This is rigorous and not for everyone.)

SIT and HIT Exercise Format

- In the High Intensity Interval Training (HIT) session — using a stationary bicycle, you ride for 2 to 4 minutes at a low cycling speed, then suddenly burst into high speed for 15 to 60 seconds, then return to the slower speed for 2 to 4 minutes, then return to the high speed for another 15 to 60 seconds, repeating this slow/ fast sequence for 30 minutes, 3 times/week, for a total of 90 minutes/week.

- In the Sprint Interval Training (SIT): again, you use a stationary bicycle, but this time — each 4.5 minute periods of low intensity cycling is split with all-out sprints lasting 30 seconds. This sequence is repeated 4 to 6 times in a 30 minute period, 3 times/week, for a total of 90 minutes/week.

These SIT / HIT sessions of 90 minutes/week were found to be as effective as other 60 minute workout sessions performed five times/week (300 minutes/week) — a true time-effective method of achieving cardio-performance.

Your Heart

Sport and exercise scientists at the Liverpool John Moores University and the University of Birmingham who performed the study believe these less time-consuming exercise methods will be suitable to improve health and will gain acceptance. Participating exercisers will appreciate the reduction in time and the improved safety such as not running along busy roadways and risking joint injury.

The 7-Minute Exercise Circuit

High Intensity Circuit Training using resistance training combined with aerobic exercise is another fitness and exercise plan developed for busy people. The Human Performance Institute, Division of Wellness and Prevention, of Orlando, Florida, was featured in a NY Times article in 2013. People who are in generally fit condition can maximize a workout in a short time period. No equipment is needed and body weight is used as resistance.

A dozen different exercises are performed for 30 seconds with a ten second break between sessions. The total circuit workout time is seven minutes and can be repeated. Although it is not recommended for people with heart trouble or high blood pressure, this short strenuous workout can provide great benefit. More information with photos of the various exercises is available at acsm-healthfitness.org. Some exercises are: jumping jacks, wall sit, plank, lunge, push-ups and step-up onto a chair.

How do people live to be 100?

In 2010, there were 131,000 people in the United States over the age of 100. By 2020, the projected number will be 214,000. The same upward trend is present in other industrialized countries. We are now tracking *super-centenarians* — people living over 110 years of age.

Centenarian studies on those reaching the age of 100 are ongoing in numerous countries. Individuals in Japan living on the Islands of Okinawa have the highest life expectancy in the world at 81.2 years. As you might imagine, people who live to be 100 are not usually overweight, nor do they smoke. In fact, they exercise their bodies and their brains. They do not look at retirement as a goal, in fact, they maintain jobs longer. Physical activity is part of their everyday routine. Working, walking, bicycling, golfing, karate and Tai Chi are combined with art, painting, playing music, reading and socializing.

In Okinawa there are 34 centenarians for every 100,000 people. In America, there are about ten people over 100 years of age for every 100,000 people, three times less.

There is a high genetic correlation with living to be this old. If your parents and grandparents lived into old age, your chances are better than if your relatives died young. However, the search is ongoing for the genetic attributes that correlate with old age. Genes are not always the whole story, although in New England, researchers may have found a key link to long life in a unique section on Chromosome 4; they found evidence of this unique area in 137 sets of very old siblings.

Axel inherited the genes for long life. If you are like Axel and fortunate enough to have been born into a family with a history of living long, you might become an octogenarian even if you don't make the best lifestyle choices. Axel and seven of his siblings lived into their 90's and beyond. Axel out-lived all of them and celebrated his 107th birthday — and it wasn't because he was a health nut. In fact, he was known to drink alcohol in excess, loved to eat red meat, and smoked or chewed tobacco all his life, right up to the end. What he did do that may have benefited him was he stopped drinking when he retired, and after his wife died, he adopted a stray dog that came to his house one day. Axel and his beloved dog Sue were inseparable. They took walks nearly everyday until Sue died 17 years later. Axel was a thin wiry man with social charm. He found humor in life and joked with everyone he met, especially the nurses at the home where he spent the last few years of life. Near the end, he became a little unstable ambulating and chose to get around in a wheelchair. Nearly every day he managed to wheel himself outside where he enjoyed a "good chew" of tobacco. He showered and dressed without help and joined fellow nursing home residents in the dining room for meals. When family members came to visit, he enjoyed their conversation and always asked about other family members by name. One night, Axel went to bed as usual with no complaints. He had been talking earlier that day about wanting to see his oldest sister who had preceded him in death. Axel died in his sleep. He was loved by many and blessed with good genes, a good wife, a loving pet and living an active physical and social life.

Many studies correlate longer life and less depression in those who have pets. Women tend to live much longer than men. Female centenarians outnumber males 9 to 1. Women are usually more social than men and studies have found strong social ties correlate with living longer and healthier.

The Okinawa population consumes fewer calories than Americans do by 10-20%. They also eat less saturated fat, more omega-3 fatty acids (fish) and a diet consisting primarily of fresh fruits and vegetables. We will talk about longevity at length in another volume of Lipstick Logic, but for the time being, by following the Okinawan patterns of eating and activity it would help reduce your risks for heart disease.

Also, take a look at the people who live on the island of Ikaria on the Aegean Sea; and men in Sardinia, where there is the highest concentration of men over 100; or in Okinawa where women live the longest. Researchers from the University of Athens concluded the people of Ikaria are 2.5 times more likely to reach the age of 90 as US citizens. All of these cultures consume similar foods and share lifestyles. Another factor may be their isolation and mix of longevity genes producing individuals carrying traits for health and long life. Many studies are examining factors that might be related and could contribute to a better understanding of longevity traits. For now, we believe their genetics, food choices and lifestyle play a large role.

Now let's look at what to eat in more detail, food's role in body function and the methods of treatment being used most successfully today to reduce the effects of bad cholesterol.

Betty Kuffel, MD

Chapter 11
Diet Implications for Heart Health

Healthy Eating

If you have blood relatives with a history of heart attack, stroke or diabetes, you may also be at risk for those problems. If you have an inherited defect in cholesterol metabolism, it is important to seek medical attention and have a lipid panel and fasting blood glucose after having nothing to eat or drink during the 8-12 hours preceding the test. These studies will provide baseline levels to help monitor any corrective measures.

The first measure in treating elevated cholesterol or glucose levels is to consume a diet consisting of reduced saturated fats, sugars and carbohydrates. In addition to improving health through diet modification, supplements may be beneficial.

Eat the Mediterranean Cuisine – No matter where you live. You may say—*Oh, please, not another diet!* You've no doubt heard of, and maybe tried some of the many popular diets. The Atkins Diet, the South Beach Diet, Cabbage Soup Diet, Grapefruit Diet, Subway Diet or the Weight Watchers or Nutrisystem diets, and want to either laugh or scream when you think of yet another diet. Many of these fad "diets" are not sustainable. Their approaches to weight control are not something you can follow for the rest of your life.

Our objective is not to put you on a diet, but to educate you about the benefits of a heart-healthy eating plan. Years of research show populations bordering the Mediterranean Sea have a reduced incidence of heart disease. Their traditional meals incorporate fish, fruits, vegetables, grains, and low meat and meat product consumption. In addition to the right food choices, appropriate portions of food and frequent exercise are essential for weight control and health. Olive oil and an occasional glass of red wine provide additional antioxidants and resveratrol, known to be heart-healthy. If you don't drink alcohol, consider substituting dark grape or blueberry juice for similar benefits.

As advocated by Dr. Walter Willett of Harvard University School of Public Health and others in the 1990's, the "Mediterranean diet" is really based on the eating patterns

104

of the Island of Crete, Greece and southern Italy. This <u>excludes</u> some of the Mediterranean cultures where animal fat and butter consumption are prevalent. Dr. Ancel Keys, with many others, examined cardiovascular disease in many countries around the world. Their findings showed a reduction in overall cardiovascular disease and cardiovascular mortality in those consuming the Mediterranean diet limiting animal fat as described above. Dr. Keys lived on the southwest coast of Italy for many years consuming the diet he advocated and nearly reached the age of 101.

Many years have passed since 1956 when the American Heart Associated informed people that foods high in saturated fats would lead to heart disease and encouraged people to eat a low-fat diet. Not only have the healthful results of a low-fat, high fresh produce diet held true for reducing heart disease, additional studies focused on other aspects of health, found a reduction in cancer and cancer mortality, and a reduced incidence of dementia.

♥ Mediterranean Cuisine Basics:
- Eat plant-based foods: including vegetables, fruits, whole grains, legumes and nuts.
- Avoid butter. Use healthy oils such as olive oil and canola.
- Instead of salt, use herbs and spices for flavors.
- Limit red meat to less than once a week.
- Eat fish and poultry twice a week.
- Drink red wine in moderation (optional).
- Exercise (not optional).

Mediterranean lifestyle pattern also recognizes the importance of enjoying meals with companions. What's not to like about eating healthful foods with family and friends?

Although the Sonoma region of California and the Mediterranean coastal areas are on opposite sides of the earth, environmentally they are similar. People living in these regions tend to live healthier than those in other areas of the world. The indigenous Japanese who live along the ocean on Okinawa also live longer than other cultures; as do the Seventh Day Adventists who follow a plant-based food regimen. What they all have in common are food choices and lifestyle; the way they eat and live each day.

The Lipstick Logic Cardio-Action approach has proven benefit. Many people set out from time to time determined to eat healthy food and exercise, but for one reason or another fail. They fall back to old habits of snacking on chips, eating fast foods and watching too much television.

The challenge is to understand what you are doing and why. With proper knowledge, it is easier to choose a path for life by adopting a pattern of healthy eating for you and your family. Begin with young children and make positive changes leading to a longer, healthier life. For snacks, offer fruit, crunchy vegetables, yogurt or un-sugared cereal instead of gummy fruit snacks, processed meat, hot dogs, pizza and sweets.

In the cultural areas mentioned earlier, daily food choices include healthy foods such as fresh fruits, fresh vegetables, and fish, all low in fat and sugar. Exercise comes easy in the warm climates and exercise is essential to health. But, you don't have to live near the Mediterranean to reap the benefits of their lifestyle.

Have you ever noticed bright-minded, mobile 90-year-olds, who appear twenty years younger and wonder why they have the fortune of good health? It is a safe bet most of them are of normal weight and active mentally, socially and physically. They probably never smoked, but drank an occasional glass of wine. In that equation there is a combination of good choices, some good luck and good genes. **There is a strong genetic component to longevity, but you can counteract "good genes" by making bad life choices. And you can offset "bad genes" by making good choices.**

♥ *The Lipstick Logic Cardio-Action Plan is not a diet. It is a way of life.*

We are not talking about "going on a diet" as a calorie reduction plan — instead, we are encouraging you to take a new path — a path that will become a journey of a lifetime. This new journey will include appropriate sized portions of fresh food and regular exercise.

Your Heart

There are no magical foods. Nothing melts belly fat. When weight comes off, adipose tissue stored in fat cells gradually becomes less. It melts away all over the body and not from pockets here and there. Even doing many sit-ups a day, your belly will not burn off more fat selectively; only abdominal muscle tone will improve.

We are each born with a body type. Some of us put on more weight in the legs or thighs, and some predominantly gain around the waist or buttocks. Excess carbohydrate intake does not particularly result in abdominal weight gain. Triglycerides are packed into fat cells wherever they may be. As you lose weight your most prominent storage areas will be the last to go.

Weight gain and weight loss are related to body fuel requirements. If you have eaten more calories than your body needs to operate, those calories are stored as fat. If you have burned more calories than you have taken in, then the body will utilize stored fat for energy and you will lose weight. One pound gained or lost = 3500 kcal, or calories as we call them.

If you eat a 400 calorie piece of pie in addition to your energy needs, to be calorie-neutral, here is what you will have to do: If you weigh 160 pounds, walking at a rate of 2 mph, you would burn 183 calories in one hour. You will have to walk well over 2 hours to earn the pie, or you will store the excess as fat. For comparison, a medium or large milkshake adds 750-1000 calories. You must walk many miles, 4 or more, to earn the calories in that milkshake and avoid weight gain.

It doesn't matter what time of the day you eat or how much water you drink with meals. Many people believe in gimmicks. There are no gimmicks. Think about it. Did the healthy people we mentioned earlier all get together and share meal plans? No. They ate fresh foods selected from their gardens or purchased at local markets, and fresh fish from the sea. They ate little fat and very little red meat. That information provides a starting point.

By changing the way you shop, what you select when you buy groceries and the methods you use in preparation, you can make a big change in your overall eating pattern. Processed foods are more expensive than fresh foods. Switching to fresh healthful selections will cost you less.

After people complained about the cost of Mediterranean food choices, especially fish and low-fat meat, a study of food bank recipients revealed some interesting data. Changing the focus to remove foods not needed to improve health such as: meat, snacks, desserts and carbonated drinks, the choices were economical. Those in the study attended cooking classes for six weeks, using fresh fruits and vegetables along with low glycemic grains. With the increased consumption of fresh produce, their spending on food dropped, as did their reliance on the food bank. Half of the participants in the study also experienced desired weight loss.

Avoid the center aisles of your grocery store where all the packaged foods are displayed. Purchase from the dairy, meat and produce sections only. Leave all the packaged goods behind other than some healthful non-sugared cereals. That may sound frightening because the packaged goods are designed to save you time, and time is valuable. But time-saving products not only cost you more financially, they may also be ruining your health. It is a lifestyle of prosperity that is making us sick. Returning to "the basics" is the journey we advocate to help you take action today to prevent cardiac disease, obesity and possibly early death.

A study done at the University of San Francisco School of Medicine compared findings in two groups of people, those who ate their regular diet and those who ate basic components of the Mediterranean diet but excluded dairy, cereal grains and legumes. In ten days, all the health parameters we are aiming for improved: blood pressure, glucose tolerance and lipid profiles. Insulin production also decreased, while insulin sensitivity improved.

Glycemic Index (GI)

Before discussing specific foods, it is important to know something about a measurement called the *Glycemic Index*. It is a numerical scale used to indicate how fast and how high a particular food can raise blood glucose (blood sugar) level. Foods with a low glycemic index allow the body's blood glucose to creep up slowly allowing pancreatic insulin release to take effect and utilize the glucose, maintaining normal glucose levels.

Foods with a high GI cause the blood glucose to rise rapidly making it more likely glucose levels will surge and pancreatic release will lag. In Type 2 diabetics, the pancreas releases high levels of insulin but tissue has become resistant to its effects and glucose remains elevated for long periods. In diabetics, glucose spikes add to destructive inflammatory changes.

Blood Glucose Levels
- Normal fasting: less than or equal to 110 mg/dL
- Pre-diabetic: 110-125 mg/dL
- 2 hours after eating: less than 140mg/dL
- Random: 80-120mg/dL

♥ Eat foods with low glycemic indexes. This is a helpful way to begin a new journey toward healthier eating. Knowing more about low glycemic index foods is valuable for people with pre-diabetic and diabetic states, too. Choose fruits, vegetables and proteins, and *complex* carbohydrates including whole wheat products. Reduce sugar intake. **Eating high glycemic index foods raises blood glucose rapidly and stresses the pancreas.**

There are many glycemic index sources of information on reputable online sites. Dieticians and diabetic counselors are versed in the importance and can help you with food choices. Paying attention to the glycemic index and avoiding those high GI foods will help diabetics maintain a normal blood sugar.

US food nutrient labels do not indicate the GI index of foods, so you'll need to independently educate yourself more about the Glycemic Index. You can find a free index online at: naturalhealthinspector.com

In non-diabetic people, the body is able to maintain the blood sugar within a narrow range. When pancreas insulin-producing cells are constantly stressed to pour out more insulin into the blood, based on recent studies, this is what happens:
- Blood sugar rises.
- More and more insulin is necessary because tissue cells become insulin resistant.
- The pancreas fatigues and fails.
- Type 2 diabetes results.

• Medications and injected insulin become necessary to normalize blood sugar.

Metabolic processes within the body are complex and involve many essential substances, proteins, vitamins and enzymes. Entire lifetimes of study are devoted to understanding all the interactions in biochemistry. Some disease processes have been identified that are related to genetic aberration of steps in these cycles. Below are simplistic overviews of nutrients:

Nutrients
Carbohydrates/sugars: Carbohydrates are complex molecules containing various combinations of the sugars: glucose, fructose and galactose. The body acts on these molecules through very complex metabolic processes breaking them down to usable sugars. Glycogen is the glucose molecule stored in the body for energy.

Proteins: Protein molecules are made up of amino acids and are the building blocks of muscle. Many amino acids are synthesized by the body, but there are ten *essential amino acids* that must be supplied by the foods we eat. They are found in grains, legumes, nuts, meat and dairy.

Fats: Body fats contain fatty acids and glycerol; these form the building blocks of cell membranes, hormone structures and triglyceride-based storage fat used for energy.

Chapter 12
Plant-based and Mediterranean Cuisine

Overview of Diets

As we see from statistics in developed countries around the world, what we eat is killing us. Before the age of processed easy-access foods, we worked hard, gardened and ate a diet similar to those along the Mediterranean Sea and others who consume a primarily plant-based diet. Many studies have documented longer healthier lives by following the eating and lifestyles of these people.

Terminology has changed over recent years. Vegetarian is no longer the descriptor of someone who chooses not to eat meat products, instead it is *plant-based.* True plant-based eating is *vegan,* without any animal-based products: no meat, eggs or fish; and some say — no honey. Not eating honey is no big deal. There are many plant-based natural sweeteners such as maple syrup and agave to use instead of honey.

For some people, giving up meat is unthinkable. Because the Mediterranean diet is primarily plant-based with small amounts of added fish and lean meat, the cuisines will be discussed together. When you read about these diets, you will see differences and more descriptors. *Whole food plant-based* practitioners don't even allow olive oil or other plant oils because they are processed and not *whole.* Don't become neurotic about food choices. Instead, learn to make your selections with thought. We know olive oil is monounsaturated oil and has healthy benefits when consumed in small amounts, so why not use it?

Some people find the Mediterranean cuisine more appealing and easier to follow than plant-based because there are some acceptable meat options. Benefits from both include reduction in heart and vascular disease, reduction in Type 2 diabetes, better glucose control, weight loss—and longer life.

A British study which began in 1993 was recently published in the *American Journal of Clinical Nutrition.* The study included more than 44,000 people, 34% of them ate plant-based diets. Those who ate no meat had a 32% lower risk of heart disease than people who ate meat.

Omitting saturated fat and excess sodium helps to lower cholesterol and blood pressure levels. Eating a plant-based diet can be very healthy. To be healthy and plant-based, people must pay attention to their choices. Not all people living a vegetarian lifestyle are thin and healthy. Eating too much of a good thing can happen to them, too. Many gain weight related to excess portions of complex carbohydrates and grains. If you are ready to eat a plant-based diet, learn healthful choices and understand proper portions. Check out Realage.com and other reputable sites for valuable fact-based information.

You may have heard about the *paleo diet; the paleolithic diet.* It is a long way from Main Street USA; it's the *caveman diet.* It carries some of the same benefits to health as the plant-based diet and is similar to Mediterranean choices. Paleo choices include lean free-ranging animal products, game and fish but *exclude* dairy products, cereal grains, legumes, refined sugars and processed foods. Cavemen struggled to get enough food, walked everywhere and it is very unlikely they were overweight. Lack of exercise is a prime component of today's obesity problem.

The Cardio-Action Plan focuses on fresh fruits, vegetables and whole grain selections. If you choose to follow the Mediterranean cuisine, helpful details on the healthiest choices of meat and fish are included later in this section.

Transition to Plant-based Cuisine

The whole concept of not having meal plans based around meat is foreign to most people. The transition from an animal-based diet to a plant-based diet can be simplified. Many people eat eggs for breakfast. You could choose to eat them but once you transition to eating whole-grain cereal, smoothies, yogurts and fruit, it is unlikely you will want to return to your old ways. If you still want eggs, use the whites only. Egg whites are an excellent protein source and zero cholesterol if you omit the yolk.

Your Heart provides the thought processes behind healthful eating to help you make good choices and lifestyle transitions. Not only will these changes impact your health but they may improve the health of your children, family, friends and pets, once you are all involved.

To begin a plant-based diet you may not need to purchase special kitchen equipment. It is likely you have everything on hand. You'll need a few sharp knives, a blender, vegetable peeler, and a basket for steaming vegetables. Steaming is important to maintain the nutrition in cooked vegetables. A knife sharpener will be an important tool because you'll want knives sharp for vegetable preparation.

To begin, make a list of the commonly eaten meals and snacks you prefer. Then, take a look at the content of each of them and see what you could change to substitute a healthier choice. For example, if you usually eat white toast or a bagel slathered with butter or cream cheese, to make this plant-based selection healthier, use whole grain breads and instead of butter and regular cream cheese, use sugarless jam, a bit of coconut oil spread or low-fat cream cheese.

If lasagna is a favorite food, you don't have to stop eating it. Modify your lasagna recipe in the following ways: use whole-grain pasta or substitute slices of eggplant for the pasta, add tomato sauce, sliced tomatoes. spinach or other vegetables such as zucchini. Substitute usual cheeses with low fat cheese or soy products.

Soups and one-pot stews will become common in your meal plans. Once you have found some combinations you particularly like, you can alter them by making a purée and adding yet more and different colored vegetables for variety. webmd.com has some excellent plant-based and Mediterranean meal ideas.

If you particularly enjoy sweets, it may be a more difficult transition away from sugar-based food than it is away from animal products. Fresh fruits will replace sugar-laden snacks. To have something ready for a healthful snack, wash fruit and vegetables thoroughly and keep them available in the refrigerator at all times for snacks.

Whole Grains vs. Refined Grains
Whole grains are healthier. They have lower glycemic indexes than refined grains that have reduced fiber and vitamin content. Just because carbohydrates are part of these grains, it doesn't make them unhealthy. Beneficial whole grains are noted below.

Simple sugars are absorbed readily by the body and raise blood sugar, rapidly triggering insulin release by the pancreas. Carbohydrates are complex sugars the body must digest to break down their components before they can be absorbed.

Because the process takes time, elevation in blood glucose is slower than with simple sugars so insulin release is slower. This is the concept of the glycemic index of foods. Consumption of a food with a low glycemic index keeps the blood glucose on a more even level — better for everyone and essential for diabetics.

Transitioning to a plant-based or Mediterranean diet can be life-saving and weight-losing. This is very important for Type 2 diabetics. You will be cutting out all highly caloric foods and focusing on fresh fruits and vegetables. Grains are an important part of both diets, but the volume of carbohydrates and grains consumed must be thoughtful and not in excess.

Healthful whole grain products include: wheat germ, flaxseed, oat bran, rice bran, oats, wheat bran, Japanese soba noodles (made with buckwheat), hard red spring wheat (high protein content), quinoa and millet (grain-like seeds), amaranth (Aztec staple), rye, spelt (nutty flavored ancient grain), whole wheat macaroni, wild rice, buckwheat, whole grain wheat flour, durum wheat and barley.

With small differences between their glycemic indexes, it is the volume of foods you eat that really makes the difference in the calorie content of a meal and potential for weight gain. Short-grain white rice has a relatively high GI of 72 and brown rice has a GI of 55. A study in the Harvard School of Public health investigated eating white rice vs. brown rice related to the risk of developing Type 2 diabetes. Data analyzed from a lifestyle and diet questionnaire answered by nearly 200,000 people revealed eating brown rice instead of white rice decreased diabetic risk. Brown rice adds fiber more nutrients and is absorbed more slowly thus reducing blood glucose spikes.

Comparing flour ground from spelt, wheat, buckwheat and oats, you will find a volume of one cup contains about 400 calories, 80 grams of carbohydrate, and about 15 grams of protein. Mediterranean and plant-based diets include grains, so for variety, you will want to try different grains. Spelt is a species closely related to wheat and is used in breads, cereals and pastries. It is an ancient grain. Like wheat, rye, barley, triticale, kamut and farina, spelt contains gluten. Kamut is an ancient grain, high in protein with a nutty flavor and is larger than modern wheat. Farina is a cereal food made from wheat and is a rich source of iron.

Triticale is a hybrid of wheat and rye. First bred in Scotland in the 1870's, this cereal grain is grown and eaten around the world. It is grown extensively in Europe, but in the US, it is only a specialty crop.

Two more grains you will read about are emmer and einkorn, both are ancient grains. Emmer dates back to ancient tombs and is related to einkorn. Both are hardy grains that contain gluten.

Examining wheat and wheat products produces conflicting information to sort through. Many claims are not supported by controlled science-based studies. A recent best-selling book written by cardiologist Dr. William Davis, recommended stopping consumption of all wheat products because of the uniquely bad dietary characteristics of wheat resulting from its alteration by growers.

Wheat is a staple food across the world. There is no genetically engineered wheat sold in the US. Over centuries, wheat and other grains have naturally cross-pollinated, producing cross-strains. Intentional cross-pollination of wheat and rye created triticale. The grain has been sold and consumed widely for years without harm, except just like any other grain when it is eaten in excess and contributes to obesity.

Some research on wheat has been to encourage drought-resistant or disease-resistant strains to produce more food to feed hungry nations. The author, Dr. Davis, has concluded modern wheat, even whole wheat, is bad. Patients following his diet of omitting wheat have lost weight, reduced heart risks, and feel better. But, is it weight loss from calorie reduction by omitting the carbohydrate load containing wheat, or is it merely no wheat? Another theory the author has is this — changes in the wheat now produced have caused a rise in gluten sensitivity.

Gluten is not the only element in wheat that some people do not tolerate. Those with true allergies to wheat develop skin rashes that can be severe. Some develop asthma symptoms if exposed to the flour dust. However, over centuries, wheat has been a well-tolerated staple. More studies are required to prove wheat is innately harmful to those who are not gluten intolerant and do not have celiac disease.

Betty Kuffel, MD

Gluten Intolerance

Gluten intolerance is an autoimmune disease that damages intestinal villi causing the inflammatory malabsorption syndrome celiac disease. Gluten is a protein in wheat comprised of *gliadin* and *glutenin*. Related grain species containing gluten are barley, rye and triticale (the cross of wheat and rye). When the wheat protein gliadin contacts the intestine, a marked reaction occurs damaging the intestinal lining preventing the absorption of nutrients. Symptoms include intestinal cramping, discomfort, malnutrition and weight loss.

For most people, whole grains are healthful. Products eaten every day, including pasta and breads, are made with gluten-containing grains. Many people have irrationally decided to avoid gluten in their diets, thereby excluding extremely nutritious food options.

People with true gluten intolerance have *celiac disease*, also known as *celiac sprue*. In celiac disease, eating a diet free of gluten is life-saving. In the past, gluten intolerance was not easily diagnosed. Now, celiac disease is diagnosed readily with blood tests and intestinal biopsies. Proper treatment and food-choice education are readily available. Twenty years ago, this was not the case.

Some people are *gluten-sensitive or gluten-reactive*. Their tests for gluten-intolerance are normal, yet they develop diarrhea and gut cramping when they consume gluten. Stopping gluten consumption is the right action and if symptoms resolve, the person is deemed gluten-sensitive.

To be diagnosed with the celiac disease you cannot stop eating gluten and then seek medical care, you must be eating gluten when you are tested or the tests will be negative for gluten intolerance. A gluten-free diet is very restrictive and if you don't need to avoid gluten because of intestinal reactions, there is no reason to join the fad diet craze. Unless you have gluten-intolerance, a gluten-free diet is not healthier than a gluten-dense diet.

The number of people who are gluten intolerant is elusive. Some report a marked increase. The website CeliacCentral.org estimates 1% of the population experiences gluten intolerance.

Your Heart

Healthy Foods — Organic or Not?

Organic foods tend to be more costly to purchase but if you consider the fact that some commonly consumed foods are also the highest in pesticides, spending a little more for organic products may be well worth the extra money. Organic produce is grown without genetic engineering, pesticides, and synthetic fertilizers. Most foods we eat have pesticide residues on the surface. Pesticides and chemicals can also penetrate into the pulp of the fruit or vegetable, so washing doesn't remove all the danger.

♥ Washing Produce

Carefully washing food is very important to remove dirt and pesticide residue. Some produce, especially root vegetables and melons require scrubbing followed by repeated rinsing in clear water.

The University of Minnesota Extension division recommends not only washing produce under running water but adding vinegar to help kill bacteria. One easy way to cleanse smooth-skinned fruit is to saturate it with a spray containing ½ cup white vinegar + 1 ½ cups cold water. Let the foods sit for a few minutes after spraying with the vinegar solution, then rinse thoroughly and dry.

A similar method can be used for larger collections of fruits and vegetables. After cleansing the sink, place produce in the sink (or a large pan) and spray each piece to saturate it with the vinegar solution. Leave 2-3 minutes, then rinse under running water and pat dry. Three studies reported as much as 98% of bacteria were removed when using vinegar combined with thorough rinsing in cold water.

In 2002, the US Department of Agriculture instituted standards for organic food. The Environmental Protection Agency is also involved in determining risks and toxicity from exposures. Based on the Food and Drug Administration data, the following information about food safety is published by the Environmental Working Group

Highest level of pesticide residue: apples, strawberries, peaches, spinach, nectarines, grapes, sweet peppers, potatoes, blueberries, lettuce, coffee, chocolate, kale, collard greens, green beans celery.

Lowest level of pesticide residue: watermelon, bananas, onions, pineapples, mangos, avocados, sweet corn, eggplant, cabbage, kiwi, asparagus, mushrooms, domestic cantaloupe, peas, grapefruit.

Whatever the source, it is important to cleanse food thoroughly. Rinsing in cold water with vinegar is important. Whenever possible, avoid non-organic foods from the high pesticide list and purchase fresh produce from local organic farms or grow your own.

Fresh Produce
Fruit

For those who do not live in areas where fruits grow and costs are lower, shopping for in-season fruits makes sense. Take advantage of sales, and when possible, purchase from farmers' markets. Sometimes buying in bulk will cut costs considerably. If properly refrigerated, apples retain freshness for a long time.

♥ Apples are a top food choice. The old adage *"an apple a day keeps the doctor away"* is true. In a ten year study in the Netherlands on over 20,000 healthy people ages 20-65, there was a 52% reduction in stroke for those who ate the equivalent of one apple a day. Eating fresh pears was also protective. Apples and pears contain fiber and antioxidants. Other high fiber fruits include: bananas, berries, kiwi, oranges, pears and prunes.

Fruits contain natural sugar. Although we are not focusing on calories, it is helpful to know the general calorie content of common foods along with its GI number. The glycemic load in most fruit is low, making them good choices for everyone, including diabetics. But calorie intake is important and you cannot eat fruit mindlessly because fruit contains natural sugar and limitation is important in diabetics.

Vegetables

♥ Protein consumption is necessary for health because the body is unable to make ten *essential amino acids.* These proteins must be provided in the diet either through meat or plant products.

Adequate amounts of protein are required for muscle strength. Meat, fish and eggs are excellent sources. Vegetables also contain significant protein including: asparagus, cauliflower, broccoli, Brussels sprouts and corn. Beans and legumes are protein-rich and provide primary protein useable as a meat substitute in vegetarian diets. Mushrooms and tofu are also good choices.

Foods high in fiber tend to be filling and satisfy the appetite longer. The vegetables noted above are high in fiber as are: cabbage, carrots, Garbanzo beans or chick peas, spinach, mushrooms, peppers and eggplant.

Grains, Nuts and Seeds
Grains

Whole grains provide a large portion of both the Mediterranean and plant-based diet. Not only are they high in fiber, they contain antioxidants, vitamins, magnesium and iron. They are delicious, filling and can be eaten in many ways. Oatmeal, corn, whole wheat, brown rice, barley, millet, sorghum, spelt, rye and quinoa are all great choices. Even popcorn is a whole grain and a healthful low calorie snack if you omit butter and salt.

Nuts

Many nuts are delicious and good for you, but are also loaded with calories. With that said, they are still a healthful choice in small quantities. One ounce of nuts is considered a serving. One ounce of almonds (23 nuts) =160 calories. Almonds contain monounsaturated fats that help raise HDL and lower LDL. They also contain vitamin E and numerous minerals.

Overall, nuts are a healthy food choice because they contain omega 3-fatty acids, fiber and vitamin E. Walnuts contain high amounts of omega-3 fatty acids (14 half walnut pieces = 185 calories). Macadamia nuts, almonds, hazelnuts and pecans are heart healthy. Like grains, nuts are caloric and must be eaten in small quantities.

One cup of peanuts, two handfuls, contains about 800 calories. Unless you are trying to gain weight, eating a cupful of nuts is a very bad choice for snacking. Sunflower seeds, though nutritious, fall into the same category as peanuts.

A peanut butter sandwich on whole wheat bread is healthful but the calorie content precludes eating it for a snack.

It can be an entrée. A tablespoon of peanut butter, less than most people use on a sandwich, contains 100 calories. Calculation of calories in a peanut butter sandwich: bread/slice=70 calories x 2 = 140; 2 Tablespoons of peanut butter = 200 calories, 1 Tablespoon of butter = 100 calories. Total calories: 440. So, if you need to cut calories, a PB sandwich is not a good snack choice. It is better to eat an apple (about 110 calories, with 0-fat, 0-cholesterol, 2 mg sodium, 5.4 grams fiber, 23 grams sugar, vitamin A, C, calcium and iron).

Although high in calories, it is important to include some nuts in your meal plan because of the nutrition and fiber content they provide. **Almonds, pistachios and pine nuts are the lowest in calories.** Examples: 49 pistachios = 190 calories, 165 pine nuts (small and costly) = 190 calories. Macadamia nuts are about 18 calories each (11 = 200 calories). Bottom line — buy unsalted almonds. There are about 6 calories in each nut; ten almonds make a tasty and healthy snack, and only contain 60 calories.

In the long run, you can eat all of these, but in all cases, portion control is important. If you have a weight problem and would like to shed a few pounds while eating healthier, cutting back on portions is a major key to success. Eat vegetables for snacks.

Flaxseed

Flaxseed is another healthy consumable seed being added to some commercial cereal products. Flaxseeds are fed to chickens to induce higher levels of omega-3 fatty acids in their eggs and are used in ground or liquid forms as dietary supplements. The most beneficial components are the seed's omega-3s and fiber. In animal studies, flaxseed substances called lignans appear to have some cancer inhibition quality. Studies are ongoing.

♥ Olive Oil

We have discussed fats, both unsaturated and saturated. Olive oil is one of the healthy fats and a primary product of the Mediterranean. California is also a major olive producer.

Olive oil is a monounsaturated fat that can lower LDL cholesterol. It helps protect against coronary artery disease — one of the main aims of eating right. Another aspect of olive oil consumption is its protection against cancer and maintenance of brain function with aging. Consumption of 2 Tablespoons of olive oil per day correlates with increased cognition. So, it is good for your brain and your heart! If you need oil in your cooking, when possible, use olive oil.

Note: All oils contain about 100 calories per tablespoon. You might as well choose to use a healthy one.

A few olive oil facts: *Virgin olive oil* is oil obtained from a single pressing. *Extra virgin oil* is the highest quality. Because this has a delicate flavor, it is best for salads and dipping. *Fine virgin oil* is slightly less perfect but excellent. There are many other grades. *Refined* oil lacks the flavor of virgin oil. *Pure* is a blend of refined and virgin, often lower in cost. All are equally nutritious.

♥ Mediterranean Cuisine Details:
The bulk of the Mediterranean diet is composed of grains and vegetables. Much smaller quantities of protein (meat, fish, eggs, or legumes) and fruit make up the rest of the meal structure.

Dairy products, including cheese, are eaten in low to moderate amounts, as are fowl and fish. In the plant-based diet or for those intolerant to lactose, many milk substitutes are healthful and can be also be used in cooking. Many commercial products made from nuts and coconuts are delicious. For adults with lactose intolerance, try using nut milks, such as almond milk, in your coffee. Some of them are flavored and add calories so be sure to check labels.

Animal protein is not necessary to obtain adequate protein intake for health. Learning which vegetables are packed with protein will help in your decisions. High protein choices include: chick peas, nuts, tofu, beans, pumpkin, squash, tempeh (a soy food), quinoa, and sunflower seeds.

Along with the foods you choose to eat, portion size is very important. To make portion estimates easier, instead of following the old food pyramid and estimating amounts the way most of us learned at one time or another, the US Department of Agriculture (USDA) has developed a new visual—a plate divided into four parts.

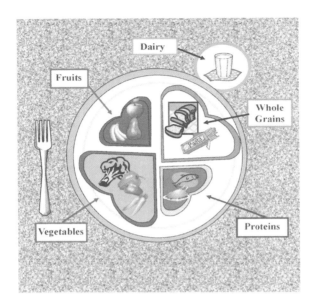

Vegetables and grains predominate. They are shown in equal allotments on the plate; two smaller portions are fruits and proteins. The dairy component is represented by a small glass of milk. This could be substituted with: a serving of low-fat yogurt, cheese, cottage cheese, low fat or almond milk.

Traditional US meals have long been based on pasta, white bread, white rice, large red meat portions (often fried) and topped off with fancy desserts or ice cream. Therefore, the whole concept of changing to a Mediterranean diet can be jarring. From experience, we know the transition isn't easy, but if you begin to think "color" when you are making food choices — it's an easy way to help get away from the typical US "white" food plan and move toward fresh plant-based foods and more salmon.

Once you begin the transition, eating two vegetables with each meal, no fried foods and stick to whole grain cereals and breads, with fruit for dessert, your old way of eating will no longer taste good. Your taste buds will soon come to reject foods like bacon, fried eggs and rare steaks, as foods not worth the health risks. You'll choose to not eat them, and not feed them to your family. After personally making the changes to eat healthier, it can take a few weeks for the smell of a greasy hamburger with fried onions to morph from "delicious" to "undesirable."

You may find it helpful to use a little self-talk and begin thinking of sausage, brats, hamburgers, chicken fried steak, Philly steak and bacon as <u>poison.</u> (A bacon cheeseburger is one of the unhealthiest choices you can make).

If you are wondering — *"What can I eat?"* At the <u>MayoClinic.com</u> website there are excellent Mediterranean recipes, as there are at many other Internet locations. Also, at the end of the book, there are a few suggested selections for breakfast, lunch and dinner.

<u>Comparing Protein Options</u>
Fish and Omega-3 Fatty Acids
From reading the information on omega-3 fatty acids, you know they help lower blood pressure and cholesterol. Omega-3s also lower triglycerides and even reduce inflammation in the body. We also know from many studies, eating fish helps to combat heart disease. Many people are not "fish-eaters," they are "meat-eaters" and don't want to change. If everyone realized eating two servings of high omega-3 fish per week would reduce their risk of dying from coronary artery disease by 36%, do you think they'd do it? One would hope.

The cost of fresh and frozen fish prevents some people from buying it, but even if you eat canned fish, you benefit as long as long as the fish is wild-caught ocean fish and not farmed. Farmed fish can be higher in pollutants including mercury and by some reports may be lower in omega-3s. Wild ocean fish are safer from both nutritional and contaminant standpoints. Twice a week consumption of 3 ounces of salmon, cod, or canned fish such as tuna, herring, anchovies or sardines will work. It is the omega-3 fatty acids in these fish that make them so nutritious.

If you hate fish, try eating canned tuna or salmon. If that doesn't work for you, fish oil supplements are beneficial, but recent reports show eating fish is the best choice.

Including flaxseed in your regular food choices adds plant-based omega-3s. Plant omega-3 is different and may not be as effective. It must be converted by the body to a more

Betty Kuffel, MD

active form to be utilized, but the large Nurses' Health Study showed benefit.

Seafood and Ocean Fish
Many fish are high in omega-3 fatty acids. Some of the highest are: salmon, tuna, sardines, anchovies and mackerel. (Note: Nutrition facts are from nutritiondata.self.com)

A report from the Cleveland Clinic states some fish particularly high in mercury should be avoided: These include: shark, swordfish, tilefish and King mackerel. Mercury may occur naturally in the water or from pollution. In the water, mercury is converted to methylmercury which is especially harmful to a fetus or young child. Nutritionists recommended pregnant and breast feeding women eat only 12-ounces of <u>safe</u> fish products per week including: wild salmon, shellfish, canned light tuna and smaller ocean fish.

For non-pregnant women just two fish meals per week show benefit. Many choices are available such as salmon, herring, mussels, trout, sardines and pollock.

<u>**Some Saltwater Options**</u>
Dungeness crab: Boiled. 3-ounces contain 346 mg omega-3s and 64 mg cholesterol. If you dip the crab meat in butter as most people do, you will lose the healthy benefit of this choice.

King crab: Boiled. 3-ounces; 390 mg omega-3s and 44 mg cholesterol (most servings are about 5 ounces).

Halibut: A 3-ounce portion of this dry white meat fish contains very high omega-3s at 1064 per serving and only 65 mg of cholesterol.

Lobster: Boiled. 1 cup — 5-ounces contain 125 mg omega-3s and 104 mg cholesterol. Avoid butter dip.

Mahi-Mahi: This fish is high in omega-3s but also contains 80 mg of cholesterol per 3-ounce serving. Mahi-mahi is a fast-growing ocean fish unrelated to dolphins even though alternate names include dolphin-fish.

Coho salmon (silver): 3-ounce serving: high in omega-3s at 990 mg, and low in cholesterol at 50 mg.

King salmon: Has similar nutritional values. Wild caught is preferable. *(Compare 990 mg omega-3s and 50 mg cholesterol to 3-ounces of lean beef round steak with only 4.5*

nani

mg of omega-3s and 60 mg of cholesterol – you can easily see why Salmon is a much healthier protein option.)

Salmon — **Canned:** One 3-ounce serving: 1427 mg of omega-3s and 37 mg of cholesterol.

Shrimp: Shrimp are a great source of protein and omega-3 fatty acids, but also contain cholesterol. One serving of about 12 large boiled shrimp (3.5-ounces) contains about 200 mg of cholesterol and only 106 calories. Many people who won't eat fish will eat shrimp. Even kids seem to like shrimp. The recommended daily intake of cholesterol is less than 300 mg. As a comparison, one large egg contains 186 mg of cholesterol (in the yolk). So you make your choice - one egg or a dozen shrimp?

An article published in the *American Journal of Clinical Nutri*tion reported steamed shrimp (not deep fried) are safe in heart-healthy diets. This study by researchers at the Rockefeller University and Harvard evaluated people without lipid problems to evaluate the effect of eating shrimp on their cholesterol levels. Over a nine week period each participant in the study ate three different diets, a total of three weeks each. The diets were: a baseline diet without shrimp (107 mg of cholesterol per day); a baseline diet plus shrimp (590 mg of cholesterol per day) and a baseline diet plus eggs (580 mg per day).

This review is important because for years, eating shrimp was not recommended on a heart-healthy diet. However, the following findings provide important information. Even though the number of people tested was small, the results appear valid:

- Both shrimp and egg diets raised LDL (bad) concentrations; eggs were worse, raising LDL by up to 10.2%.
- The shrimp diet also raised the LDL, but raised the HDL more than the LDL. Even though the LDL went up, the ratio remained favorable. So cardiovascular risk was not impacted based on the numbers.
- The shrimp diet lowered triglyceride levels significantly when compared to the other two diets.

Their analysis is: the favorable omega-3 fatty acid content of shrimp contributed to the lower triglyceride and higher HDL levels.

♥ Bottom line: Boiled shrimp are heart healthy food choices, so feel good about eating them. If they are not fried, shrimp are an excellent protein choice.

Scallops: Boiled mollusks: low calorie, low omega-3s and low cholesterol. This is a fine protein choice with 300 mg omega-3s/3-ounces and 45 mg cholesterol.

Smelt: These tiny fish are very high in omega-3s at 830 mg in a 3-ounce serving with 75 mg cholesterol.

Smelt are small bony fish often netted along fresh water coast lines and in the Great Lakes. Most species live at sea but breed in fresh water.

Tuna — Fresh: 3-ounce portion of fresh tuna is very high in omega-3s and low in cholesterol; 1414 mg of omega-3s and 40 mg of cholesterol.

Tuna — Canned: 3-ounces is usual portion. 6-ounce can: 818 mg omega-3s and 36 mg cholesterol.

Freshwater Fish

Many of these fish have lower omega-3s and higher cholesterol content than the ocean fish. However, comparing them to hamburger, steak and pork, freshwater fish are a fine protein choice.

Bass — mixed species: A good choice; 3-ounce serving contains 378 mg of omega-3s and 31mg of cholesterol.

Catfish: A 3-ounce serving is high in omega-3s at 464 mg and 50 mg of cholesterol. Catfish are farmed, very popular and a relatively inexpensive choice of fish. This fish is often served fried. To reduce fat calories, it is best eaten broiled or grilled.

Northern Pike: About a 3-ounce serving contains low 170 mg omega-3s and 46 mg of cholesterol.

Perch (mixed species): This is a plentiful little fish. About 3 ounces/two fillets contain 300 mg omega-3s and 100mg cholesterol.

Tilapia: Tilapia is a freshwater fish, usually farm-raised and has low levels of mercury. Less expensive than most fish, they have lower omega-3s. A 3-ounce serving: 205 mg of omega-3s, 49 mg of cholesterol. Because of the lower omega-3 content, many studies have been done to evaluate the usefulness of adding flaxseed to provide increased omega-3 fatty acids to the fish's diets. Even if the omega-3s are lower than salmon, this is still a good source of healthy low-fat protein.

Trout (rainbow, wild): Many varieties; 3-ounce serving: high in omega-3s (1000 mg); cholesterol per serving is 60 mg.

Walleyed Pike: A 3-ounce fillet is relatively high with 430 mg omega-3s and 102 mg cholesterol.

Meat and Poultry

Meat choices must be boneless, all fat trimmed and broiled/baked or boiled to decrease consumption of unhealthy saturated fats/cholesterol.

Bacon: This food is not on the Lipstick Logic list of healthy choices because of the high calorie, high sodium and high saturated fat content. Turkey bacon is not a good choice either, for the same reasons.

Beef: Top Sirloin, fat removed, 6-ounces, broiled: 28 mg omega-3s, 100 mg cholesterol, 320 calories.

Beef: Ground chuck (Hamburger - 80% lean/20% fat), 3 ounces, broiled; 15 grams fat, 77 mg cholesterol, 230 calories (fat calories 137). Note: Most hamburger servings are larger than 3 ounces. ("Half-pounder" = 8 ounces = 613 calories + 1 slice (1 ounce) cheddar cheese 113 calories = 726 calories, just for the meat and cheese. Add two buns and mayo and it's close to 1000 calories.) Add bacon and it's even more.

Pork Loin: Boneless, lean with all fat removed, 3-ounces, broiled: 8.5 mg omega-3s and 78 mg cholesterol.

Game Meat

Bison: 6-ounce broiled lean 1 inch thick steak: 54 mg omega-3s, 141 mg cholesterol, 317 calories.

Elk: broiled, lean, 6-ounce steak: 35 mg omega-3s, 90 mg cholesterol, 200 calories.

Moose: roast, 6-ounces, lean: 64 mg omega-3s, 164 mg cholesterol, 290 calories.

Venison: 6-ounce broiled lean 1 inch thick steak: 44 mg omega-3s, 130 mg cholesterol 243 calories.

Poultry

Turkey, roasted, dark meat: 5 ounces: 238 mg omega-3s, 120 mg cholesterol, 262 calories.

Turkey, roasted, breast meat: 5 ounces: 196 mg omega-3s 103 mg cholesterol, 265 calories.
Chicken, roasted, dark meat: 5 ounces: 252 mg omega-3s, 130 mg cholesterol 287 calories.
Chicken, roasted, breast meat: 5 ounces: 98 mg, omega-3s 119 mg cholesterol 231 calories.

Animal-based Protein Choices:
The benefits of eating a Mediterranean cuisine, low in red meat and low in saturated fat, have been known for years. Eating less red meat is important because of the known cardiovascular disease risks. Saturated fat is part of this equation, but recently, researchers at the Cleveland Clinic revealed *carnitine* plus intestinal bacteria may be part of the real cause for atherosclerosis related to eating red meat.

Carnitine is a protein derivative produced in the body and is contained in meat and dairy products. Research revealed bacteria in the digestive tract of meat eaters metabolized and changed carnitine into a harmful product called TMAO (trimethylamine N-oxide) that promotes atherosclerosis. Comparison of meat-eaters, vegetarians and vegans showed marked differences. After eating large amounts of carnitine, plant-based eaters did not produce much TMAO; meat eaters did.

When the blood level of TMAO is high, risk for atherosclerosis rises. Researchers are now focusing on how intestinal bacteria may be the actual mechanism for accelerated atherosclerosis in meat eaters because of the type of intestinal bacteria they carry. As more research is published, we may find better correlation with specific guidelines for meat consumption.

There are many forms of carnitine used in metabolic pathways in the body. Research done by the Mayo Clinic analyzing the L-carnitine form, found its use highly favorable in the setting of an acute heart attack. Metabolic pathways in damaged heart muscle are depleted of L-carnitine, a molecule required by many healthy cell mechanisms. An over-the-counter supplement was deemed safe and useful in reducing mortality, angina, rhythm problems and the size of heart muscle damage. Until more studies provide sound information for use of carnitine in sports drinks and supplements, it appears prudent to only use carnitine under the guidance of your heart doctor.

In the Mediterranean diet, along with minimal red meat, there are few eggs. We know the high cholesterol content of eggs is located in the yolk. The yolk of one large egg is 186 mg of cholesterol. Dietary cholesterol should be less than 300 mg/day. The white is high protein and very low calorie; only 16cal/large egg. You can continue to eat eggs but toss out the yolks. Don't even cook them for your pets as they, too, can become obese and develop heart disease. Egg white omelets are available in most restaurants. Even McDonald's serves egg-white Mc Muffins, just discard the meat and cheese.

♥ **<u>Plant-based protein choices</u>**: Legumes and beans are protein-rich and provide the primary protein used as a meat substitute in vegetarian diets. Broccoli, corn, Brussels sprouts, cauliflower, asparagus, soy beans/tofu and mushrooms are good choices. Also include: chick peas, nuts, pumpkin, squash, tempeh (a soy food), quinoa, and sunflower seeds.

Chapter 13
Heart Healthy Antioxidants and Supplement Overview

The Mediterranean diet is correlated with an overall reduction in cardiovascular disease risk. The eating pattern and lifestyle promote long life and good health. Many people wonder about the benefits of adding supplements to a health regimen. The following information will help you decide if you are going to spend money on something that may or *may not* provide any health improvement.

Many of these products are expensive. And, just because they are non-prescription and "natural" that does not make them safe or effective. There are many options. We will only cover a few common products showing some evidence-based value.

Antioxidants: What are they and why do we care?
When we talk about food supplements, vitamins and some food additives, the term *antioxidant* comes up and is often coupled with *beneficial.* Antioxidants are good. To understand how antioxidants combat cellular damage we need to take you along a short but meandering path of chemistry and metabolism. (Skip the next few paragraphs if you are not interested in how antioxidants work.)

Understanding Free radicals
Cells in the body are composed of many molecules. Molecules consist of atoms joined by chemical bonds. In an atom the nucleus contains positively charged protons, and neutrons with no charge. Electrons are negatively charged subatomic particles orbiting around the nucleus in shells. If a shell is unfilled then an electron is unpaired (*forming a free radical*).

So, think of *free radicals* as molecular terrorists. Simplistically, they are atoms or groups of atoms with an unpaired electron making them unstable and reactive. While scavenging other atoms to add an electron to stabilize itself, electrons are robbed from other atoms resulting in more free radicals and possibly causing cell damage leading to cancer, heart disease and aging.

Free radicals are used in some enzyme functions and are used by the immune system to destroy viruses and bacteria.

But in excess, they can damage cell protein structure and DNA causing mutations leading to cancer.

The body absorbs nutrients from food, and through oxidation, produces energy. In this process, free radicals are also released. Exposure to toxic environments, such as radiation and smoke, increases free radicals in the body. A diet high in fat produces free radicals through increased oxidation.

Antioxidants
To combat molecular "terrorists," we feed them antioxidants which supply electrons to neutralize the free radicals. **Many foods are high in antioxidants: grains, nuts, fruits, vegetables, some meats and fish.**

Free radical cell damage is implicated in heart disease, DNA mutation, aging and cancer. Because aging cells generate more free radicals which further damage cell structure, we'd like to stop them from being produced. Active enzyme systems and numerous vitamins are antioxidants. Vitamins E, C and beta-carotene are antioxidants found in many foods — in particular: fish oils, grains, citrus, cabbage-related veggies and eggs. Numerous online sources and nutrition books provide broad information on antioxidant nutrients.

A ten year study on 32,000 women, found those who ate diets highest in antioxidants had the lowest risk for heart disease. What you eat clearly makes a difference. Choices typical of the Mediterranean diet are most beneficial including fruits, vegetables, and whole grains with high antioxidant content.

BEVERAGES
Beer
Beer's rich potent antioxidant activity is from a prime ingredient called hops. In small amounts, wine and beer carry benefits, but in excess, alcohol consumption carries high risks for hypertension, heart toxicity and a myriad of health problems.
♥ Coffee
Coffee exportation is a $20 billion dollar industry. After crude oil, coffee is the most sought commodity in the world. Coffee is good for you, but like everything else you do, also drink coffee in moderation. Numerous studies show a

reduction in Type 2 diabetes in those who drink either caffeinated or decaffeinated coffee. In one study of about 193,000 people, those who drank 6-7 cups a day were 35% less likely to develop Type 2 diabetes than those who drank less than two cups a day. Even drinking 4-6 cups per day appears to lower the risk of diabetes.

Freshly brewed coffee contains antioxidants. Minerals including magnesium and chromium in coffee are involved in insulin function. Lowering risk for diabetes reduces the risks for both heart attack and stroke. In addition to all of the above benefits, there are clear links to decreased risk of Parkinson's disease and Alzheimer's dementia in coffee drinkers.

Two studies showing favorable effects from coffee consumption are the long-term study on 83,700 nurses enrolled in the Nurses' Health Study which showed a 20% lower risk of stroke in those who drank 2 or more cups per day over non-coffee drinkers. In another study on 130,000 people who drank 1-3 cups per day, they found that 20% were less likely to be hospitalized for heart rhythm issues than nondrinkers.

One would think the stimulant effect of coffee would be detrimental because caffeine can stimulate adrenaline and raise blood pressure. Some clinical studies find too much caffeine can set you up for high blood pressure, high blood sugar, and decreased bone density—not to mention jangled nerves, but let's examine some of the findings related to these claims.

Caffeine's stimulant effect can temporarily raise blood pressure but does not cause hypertension. Studies examining glucose variations with coffee report variable effects. *Improved insulin sensitivity* and improved glucose levels are associated with long term consumption of 5 or more cups of coffee per day. A short-term study comparing 2-4 weeks of coffee consumption, with those drinking no coffee, showed evidence of *increased insulin resistance* and elevation of glucose. These two results are in conflict with one showing improved insulin sensitivity and the other showing increased insulin resistance. In any case, high coffee consumption is not advocated to lower blood glucose. Long term trials measuring caffeine and coffee effects on glucose metabolism and insulin sensitivity are needed before any judgment can be made.

Coffee is a mild diuretic and affects calcium by increasing the amount of calcium and magnesium lost in the urine. One investigator stated that more than 300 mg/day of brewed coffee (about 18 ounces) accelerated bone loss in menopausal women.

One downside to coffee is the substances you add. Plain black coffee has fewer than ten calories. Add a teaspoon of sugar and you have added 23 calories. Adding half and half or liquid non-dairy creamer increases the calorie content by 50. Check the calories of what you add and see if you want to spend daily calories that way or learn to drink it black. Some coffee specialty drinks contain as much as 500 calories, a meal in itself. Also, if you are having daily barista coffee drinks, these hidden calories can jeopardize weight control goals and are expensive.

If you look around, you may find a new coffee drink made from coffee plant leaves. A recent article in the Canberra Times reported an *Annals of Botany* publication stated that *Coffea Arabica* leaves have higher levels of antioxidants, thought to be beneficial in combating heart disease, diabetes and even cancer. Coffee plant leaf tea is currently available in some health food stores.

Symptoms of excess caffeine consumption are: insomnia, tremors, nausea, vomiting, chest pains, and palpitations, among others. Practice moderation in all things.

♥ Black and Oolong Tea

A healthy aspect from the *Carnellia sinensis* plant (Black and Oolong tea source) is the content of bronchodilators. If you know someone with asthma, you may want to tell them about the benefits of these two teas. Theophylline and theobromine in the teas act on the lungs by relaxing tight airways, allowing better airflow. Tea can help calm a cough in mild lung conditions.

♥ Green Tea

Benefits of drinking green tea have been touted for years. Does this mean a confirmed coffee drinker should acquire a taste for tea? Maybe; it sounds uninteresting and if it is calorie-free, how good can it be?

Green tea contains micronutrients called catchins. These are antioxidants that scavenge the free radicals. An animal study at McGill University in Montreal on one component of the catchins, found it effective in treating prostate tumors.

Human studies are hopeful. In the lab, the green tea substance inhibits cancer growth and kills abnormal cells.

In a study involving 500 Japanese women with breast cancer, those who drank increased amounts of tea before and after surgery had lower cancer recurrence. Another cancer that may be suppressed by green tea is lung cancer. Twenty-two studies showed drinking two cups of green tea (not black) resulted in an 18% decrease in developing lung cancer. If you are already a tea drinker, but it isn't *green,* give it a try.

Some studies show green tea aids in weight loss, reduces LDL cholesterol, lowers blood pressure and relaxes blood vessels improving heart health.

If all these positive aspects of tea haven't convinced you to drink a couple of cups a day, maybe this will: green tea suppresses bacteria in the mouth and GI tract and may not only combat tooth decay, but also helps infectious diarrhea. Because of the medicinal aspects of green tea, lotions and bath salts are including green tea extracts and prescripted green tea ointments are being used to help clear warts!

♥ Grape Juice, Wine – Resveratrol

Grape juices, including red wine, contain antioxidants. But more important, they are a source of resveratrol. This is a plant compound called a polyphenol which may help reduce risks for coronary heart disease.

Research suggests resveratrol:
- Reduces inflammation
- Reduces clotting that may lead to heart attacks
- Protectively stops LDL oxidation
- Reduces insulin resistance

It also appears resveratrol activates a body mechanism that protects against a broad spectrum of weight and age-related disease. Overall, resveratrol looks beneficial but is not FDA regulated. Side effects are limited but there is some interaction with blood-thinners.

Resveratrol sources are: the skin of red grapes, blueberries, bilberries, cranberries, and peanuts. Pomegranates are a healthy antioxidant polyphenol source but do not contain resveratrol.

Your Heart

Research for resveratrol effects have been primarily animal studies. Mice fed the product live longer, are thinner with less heart disease and diabetes. Some studies show reduction in inflammatory changes and blood clotting, too. The problem is, natural products contain very small amounts and effective natural dosing is not possible. There are many costly resveratrol supplements available.

FOODS
♥ Chocolate
Chocolate contains powerful antioxidants which are *flavonoid* compounds—the same antioxidants found in fruits, vegetables and many drinks. Drs. D. R. Buhler and Cristobal Miranda and at Oregon State University have found evidence that flavonoids fight against: viral infection, allergies, clotting, inflammation, tumors and oxidants. They are also important in *slowing* the progression of dementia.

We are focused on heart health and many studies also show significant benefits in the reduction of heart disease from eating more flavonoids. That is not to say a diet of chocolate, alone, is the answer! However, a recent study showed eating dark chocolate on a daily basis reduced heart attacks and strokes. *Dark chocolate could help prevent heart problems in high-risk people.*

This study is important because they only chose people at high risk for CVD who had hypertension and metabolic syndrome. Participants who ate darker chocolate (60-70%) on a daily basis rather than milk or white chocolate lowered their risks.

Other large studies found both blood pressure reduction and improved insulin sensitivity in dark chocolate eaters. In summary, seven studies of over 100,000 people found there was a beneficial link to marked reduction in CVD and stroke, 37% and 29% respectively. Calories are of concern. Increased calories, weight gain, development of diabetes and heart disease as a result would negate the benefit. So, like everything else, eat in moderation. If you like chocolate, choose the dark variety.

Garlic
Some people would not consider eating garlic or taking supplements made from garlic because of the unpleasant smell,

bad breath and uncomfortable intestinal side effects. There are odorless/tasteless supplements, but most studies are based on garlic consumed as a food, both cooked and raw.

The National Center for Complementary and Alternative Medicine supported a large study on the safety and effectiveness of three garlic preparations. Examining blood cholesterol levels, they found no beneficial effect. This study evaluated: aged garlic extract tablets, dried powdered garlic tablets and fresh garlic.

That is not to say garlic has no value, in fact this edible bulb from a plant in the lily family has been used for medicinal purposes since the time of the pharaohs. The most common traditional uses have been for prevention of GI cancer, heart disease, high blood pressure and high cholesterol. What does science have to say?

- Atherosclerosis may be slowed.
- A long-term study showed no reduction in stomach cancer.
- A slight lowering of blood pressure in people with hypertension was found.
- Some studies have shown evidence garlic may lower some cancer risks.
- Evidence for its use to improve health is lacking.

♥ Fiber

Fiber is the indigestible parts of plants we eat. There are two types of fiber, one is soluble, and the other is insoluble. Both are equally important. Fiber does not contain nutrition but is very important as it passes through the intestines. When you consume high fiber foods such as oatmeal, lentils, fruit and vegetables, the nutrition is absorbed and the fiber is not. Insoluble fiber adds bulk to the diet and helps prevent constipation. To add more insoluble fiber, eat whole grains, bran, green beans, and leafy vegetables, along with fruit and vegetables with skins.

Soluble fibers attract water and form a gel which slows digestion, makes you feel full and slows stomach emptying. Soluble fibers help lower bad LDL and improve insulin function. Oatmeal is soluble and provides a great start for your day as an inexpensive, low-sugar healthy breakfast.

Margarine vs. Butter

One tablespoon of butter contains 15 mg of cholesterol. Margarines may be better than butter, but not all of them. We are looking for "good fats" to lower cholesterol intake. Margarine contains no animal fat; it is made from vegetable oils so it sounds healthier. The real problem is solid margarines contain the harmful trans fat.

Stick margarines contain more trans fat than soft tub margarines. Trans fats raise cholesterol just like saturated animal fats and because they also lower HDL, they raise heart disease risks. Most of us eat some form of spread every day, so making a healthful choice can impact your life and the lives of your family members. Limiting grams of fat intake is also very important from both calorie and heart standpoints. A tablespoon of oil is approximately 100 calories and 14 grams of fat.

♥ Alternative Spreads

If your cholesterol is elevated and you choose to eat margarine, purchase soft or liquid products – those without trans fats. Some fortified margarines such as **Benecol** and **Promise** help reduce cholesterol levels. Benecol, developed in Finland, is made from a natural plant component called a stanol. The European Commission reported that by consuming about 2 grams of the Benecol plant stanol/day LDL cholesterol can drop 7-10% in 2-3 weeks. Cholesterol is lowered by its action in the intestine — reducing the amount of cholesterol absorbed from food. Stanol also affects the reabsorption of cholesterol from bile. Promise is a similar product. Both have reduced fat and reduced calories. Benecol is also available as a chewable supplement.

♥ Soy

Soy protein contains plant-based estrogen-like substances called phytoestrogen. In animal studies, benefits were small, but there was reduction in cholesterol when soy protein was used as a meat substitute. It is believed that the higher intake of soy by Asian populations contributes to their lower incidence in overall cardiovascular disease when compared with a Western population.

A downside of increased consumption of soy products is the production of phytoestrogen which could enhance the growth of estrogen-positive cell type breast cancers.

The Nutrition Committee of the American Heart Association states soy substitution in the diet does not appear to provide important health benefits nor are the isoflavone supplements effective in reduction of cardiovascular disease. However, substituting soy protein for foods high in saturated fat is helpful.

SUPPLEMENTS
♥ CoQ10

This supplement has other names: Coenzyme Q10, Ubiquinol. Produced by the body, CoQ10's function is complex and necessary for cell function. Levels decrease with age and are low in heart conditions, cancer, diabetes and many chronic diseases. Some of its effects are: small decreases in blood pressure, possible slowing of dementia. Studies also suggest improvements in both angina and asthma when added to effective therapies. CoQ10 is recommended by oncologists for patients requiring chemotherapy known to be toxic to the heart often used to treat breast cancer and lymphoma. But this and a long list of uses do not have proven value.

♥ Many conditions may be helped CoQ10, but further study is needed. When supplements are consumed, CoQ10 levels rise in the body, but there was no measurable benefit shown until a recent Danish report from the 2013 European Society of Cardiology Heart Failure Association annual meeting. **A multicenter randomized double blinded study showed CoQ10 decreased all cause mortality by 50% when used in heart failure patients**. This application looks very favorable for people who are diagnosed with heart failure.

Another positive finding is–there appears to be some benefit in reducing risk of *statin myopathy*, the muscle pain sometimes seen with lipid lowering drugs. Side effects of CoQ10 are both positive and negative. They include fatigue, lower blood glucose, lower blood pressure and gastrointestinal symptoms. CoQ10 can interact with other medications including blood thinners and should only be used under the guidance of your physician.

♥ D - Vitamin

Deficiency in vitamin D places you at risk for weak bones, and at high risk for heart disease. Research released by the University of Copenhagen and the Copenhagen University

Hospital involving 10,000 Danish people showed a 64% higher risk of heart attack and a 57% higher risk of early death correlated with a low serum blood test of vitamin D. They compared very low blood levels of vitamin D, below 15 nanomols per liter, with the recommended level of 50 nm/l or greater.

People who live in northern climates and have little sun exposure tend to have lower vitamin D levels. This is because of the loss of natural vitamin D conversion due to lack of skin exposure to sunshine. To be safe, at your next physician check, ask for a vitamin D blood level. Beware of taking excessive vitamin D because it is a fat soluble vitamin and toxicity from too much is possible. Dosing is related to need and is based on monitoring the blood level.

♥ Fish Oil

In the past, many clinical studies evaluating diets rich in omega-3 fatty acids, the active substance found in oily fish, found a reduction in cardiovascular events.

The most recent Italian study of note, on fish oil supplements evaluating over 12,000 people *who already had significant risk factors* including diabetes and high cholesterol but without a myocardial infarction history, showed no benefit from taking fish oil supplement. The people were followed over a five year period. There are many studies showing benefit in other ways, especially when started prior to developing significant risk states.

In 1,800 men without clinical heart disease those with the highest intake of fish oils had a 44% lower incidence of coronary events after ten years when compared to those with the lowest intake. Eating ocean-caught, non-farmed salmon is safest and appears the most beneficial.

A meta-analysis of 16,000 patients in eleven studies, comparing placebo with a diet rich in omega-3 fatty acids and omega-3 fatty acid supplements, showed a reduction in fatal heart attacks, sudden death and total mortality. In this study there was no difference between dietary and supplement fish oils.

So, once again, we have conflicting reports over benefits. There was no evidence of harmful effects. Fish oil is an antioxidant and may be helpful for that reason alone.

Fish oil supplements can cause nausea, bloating, diarrhea and a fishy aftertaste. There is no evidence fish oil worsens diabetes control from a review of 26 trials. Special precautions are advised for people who have high triglycerides (hypertriglyceridemia) — they need to consult their personal physicians before beginning fish oil supplements.

With the recent report, at this time the experts are telling us to not bother taking fish oil supplements for heart health. Instead, eat a heart healthy diet including fish. Heart protective effects are seen with two servings of boiled or broiled fish per week.

♥ **Krill Oil**

Krill oil appears beneficial. Krill are tiny shrimp-like ocean animals and are a food supply for major species including whales, seals and sea birds. Harvesting could impact those ecosystems. There is no established standard dose or treatment recommendation available, but this supplement source may prove valuable to humans.

Like fish oil, some studies have found evidence krill oil reduces inflammation and lowers levels of the inflammation marker C — Reactive Protein. Krill oil also improves cholesterol levels, blood glucose and lowers triglycerides. Beware; the supplement interacts with many medications, especially blood thinners and other supplements. Few side effects are reported. If you are interested in exploring its use, check with your medical practitioner and watch for newly reported studies documenting safety and efficacy.

Red Yeast Rice Extract

The use of red yeast rice dates back to 800 A.D. A publication from the Ming Dynasty era (1368-1644) details a description of its use for stomach problems and circulation. If you are taking supplements, you need to understand what you are taking to be certain it is safe, and to know if there is documented evidence that it is beneficial. With the long history of its usefulness, red yeast rice extract has been shown to be effective.

The unusual yeast grows on rice and contains monacolins which block cholesterol synthesis. One of the monacolins is the active ingredient of lovastatin (Mevacor), a statin drug. Because of this, you must realize **side effects of red yeast rice extract are the same as those for statin drugs and can be**

serious. This supplement can interact with many medications and cause side effects that include: muscle and joint pain, liver damage, upset stomach, rash, dizziness and elevated blood glucose.

This product is unregulated and effective dosing is unknown. Studies need to be done to confirm its effectiveness in lowering cholesterol and its potential benefit to diabetics. At this time, experts suggest the use of tested prescription drugs over red yeast rice extract.

Algae Extract- *not yet available but being tested*

Researcher Smiti Gupta, PhD, at Wayne State University has recently released information from her animal study on treating lipid problems with algae extract. In her study, a liquid extract given to hamsters raised their HDLs. A low HDL correlates with heart disease, so raising it should be beneficial. This is exciting news as raising the good cholesterol, HDL, isn't as easy as lowering bad cholesterol components. Long-term animal studies must be done before testing begins in humans. The actual mechanism requires more study. Watch for more news on this topic.

Chapter 14
Lipstick Logic Cardio-Action Plan

Cardio-Action to Improve Health

Your Heart has provided broad evidence-based information to show the impact of heredity, lifestyle and diet on cardiovascular health. There is no perfect way to prevent and reduce the impact of heart disease. Each of us carries different genes and environmental risks, but emerging evidence shows adoption of the following Cardio-Action Plan will help improve your chances of living a healthier, longer life:

Cardio information - Know the cardiovascular history in your family, tabulate your personal heart risk factors. Include: blood glucose, blood pressure, lipid levels (total cholesterol, LDL, HDL, fasting triglyceride)— normalize your numbers, and if necessary, take medication.

Action choices – Use no tobacco. Eat a healthful diet: low in salt, low in sugar, low in bad fats (saturated and trans fats), higher in mono & polyunsaturated fats, omega-3 fatty acids; high in fiber (oats, bran, whole wheat breads, apples); keep your weight down; limit alcohol; see your physician and check labs for silent diseases.

Plan for fitness — live a mentally, socially and physically active life; include daily exercise. Surround yourself with positive friendships. Stimulate your mind and learn something new everyday.

While changing the way you eat and cook also decide what exercise you can do every day to add this essential component to your life journey. Even walking thirty minutes per day is a start. If you can't leave the house or the weather is bad, consider exercising with some of the televised exercise programs or purchase an exercise DVD that inspires you. You don't need costly exercise equipment.

A good pair of tennis shoes will take you miles toward good health as long as you put your feet in them and walk regularly.

Your Heart

INFORMATION REVIEW
Major RISK Factors:

High blood pressure
Cigarette smoking, tobacco use
High LDL cholesterol
High triglycerides
Low HDL cholesterol
Obesity, Diabetes, Metabolic Syndrome
Low activity level
Heredity Factors
Alcohol, Marijuana, Cocaine, Meth and MDPV
High levels of calcium supplements

Blood Pressure Control:

Blood Pressure readings include two numbers – the upper number is the Systolic (when the heart contracts); the bottom number is the Diastolic (when the heart relaxes and fills). The American Heart Association established three levels to gauge if your blood pressure is in a normal, pre-hypertension or hypertension range.

American Heart Association Classifications at 18 years of age and older:

Normal blood pressure is: 120/80 mm/Hg
Pre-hypertension is: 120 to 139/ 80 to 89 mm/Hg
Stage 1 Hypertension is: 140 to 159/ 90 to 99 mm/Hg
Stage 2 Hypertension is: 160+/100+ mmHg
Note: American Diabetic Association goal is less than a 140 mmHg systolic

Lipid Goals:

Total Cholesterol goal is 200 mg/dL or below.
LDL of 100 to129 mg/dL – If you have cardiovascular disease, the LDL goal is 70 mg/dL.
HDL of 60 mg/dL or higher – Higher is better.
HDL needs improvement if HDL is below 40 mg/dL in men or below 50 mg/dL in women.
Triglyceride goal is 150 mg/dL or below.

Betty Kuffel, MD

Meal Suggestions
Breakfast Choices
Be creative. Come up with healthy combinations that include whole grains, fruits and vegetables:
- Oatmeal, cooked with a few raisins and apple slices.
- Uncooked oatmeal, ½ cup plain yogurt and fruit such as blueberries, sprinkled with flaxseed.
- Cooked steel-cut oats, add fruit.
- Fruit salad without additives or with plain low-fat yogurt, whole grain toast.
- Whole grain cereal without added sugar, low fat or nut milk, and fruit.
- Whole grain bread with poached egg and fruit (egg yolk removed).
- Whole grain bread toasted with low-sugar jam, glass of low fat or nut milk, fruit.
- Three eggs scrambled (discard the yolks). Add vegetables such as spinach or asparagus.
- Three boiled eggs, no yolks, sliced tomato, fruit, and whole grain toast.

Note: Read labels on cereals and granola products. Avoid those with sugar and honey.

Lunch Choices
Many variations of salads are the easiest because ingredients can be prepared ahead of time: Rinse produce in cold water with added white vinegar. Drain thoroughly and store in a zip-lock bag or covered container in the refrigerator. Prepare carrots, celery sticks and cucumbers ahead of time. Keep tomatoes and olives on hand.
- Find a low-calorie, low-fat salad dressing you like. Some of the flavored vinegars are excellent or you can make your own with variable additives. Start with the vinegar of your choice, such as rice vinegar. Add herbs or a fruit such as raspberries.
- Topping options: chopped boiled egg whites, nuts, dried fruit (raisins, cranberries), lean meat, tofu, sliced beets, peppers.
- Whole grain bread for sandwiches with flavored mustards (use minimal mayo), add plenty of cucumber slices, avocado slices, yellow banana

144

peppers, lettuce, low-fat cheese, Dijon mustard, sliced tomatoes, etc.
- Fruit for dessert, if you are satisfied, save the fruit for a snack.

Dinner Choices

Lean meat: boiled, broiled or baked.

Many options: boneless pork loin, beef sirloin or round steak, chicken breast, turkey breast, tofu. Fish: salmon, mahi-mahi, cod, tilapia, canned tuna/salmon/ sardines and shrimp.

Or, serve healthful plant-based meals:
- Sides: two vegetables, small portion whole grains such as brown or wild rice, wheat pasta.
- Salad: mixed greens, veggies and low fat dressing.
- Bread: whole wheat dipped in flavored olive oil.
- Pasta entrees: limit pasta intake; buy whole wheat. Try various cooked whole grains. Add marinara tomato sauce, mushrooms, zucchini, and chopped tomatoes.
- Add herbs, spices and citrus to change and enhance flavors: dill, oregano, sage, basil, garlic, lemon and lime juice.

Dessert ideas: Fruit, sugar-free gelatin with fresh fruit or canned fruit with no added sugar.

Beverage: Glass of red wine or grape juice, nut milk, ice tea, tea, coffee or water.

Daily water: Intake for most adults should be at least 2 quarts. Enhance water with citrus slices, cucumber slices or fresh mint leaves.

Many colorful Mediterranean and plant-based recipes are available at MayoClinic.com.

Chapter 15
Reversal of Atherosclerosis

Overview

Coronary artery disease develops over many years. Reversal of the disease may also take years of dedicated healthy behavior, but improvements have been evident within months. It is possible to reduce cholesterol-filled arterial plaques. To begin, start with the summarized details in the preceding Cardio-Action Plan.

The following information includes the science behind the process proven to shrink plaques that cause obstruction inside arteries. With a healthful diet and statin medications, the disease won't disappear, but the plaques inside arteries impeding blood flow shrink and allow more blood to pass and supply your tissues. There is hope for improvement even if you have already been diagnosed with heart and vascular disease.

When someone hears *you have coronary artery disease*, it is usually frightening. Some people feel helpless, as if given a death sentence. Others face the diagnosis head-on and make lifestyle changes and better food choices. Inflammation and abnormal lipid metabolism are the invading enemies. Take control and mount your personal attack.

If you have been diagnosed with coronary artery disease, have had a heart attack, stroke or problems with arterial circulation anywhere in your body, the information in *Your Heart* provides a pathway to help you make changes to improve health. **If you have stents resulting in improved blood flow, you have been given a second chance. Stents are crisis interventions. They provide temporary solutions. Unless you make changes to prevent further plaque buildup, the same disease will evolve within the stent.**

Once stents are in place, they are permanent. The cells lining the artery, *endothelial cells,* grow inside and cover the stent making it part of the arterial wall. The amazing process results in a smooth surface and unobstructed blood flow. Like the original artery, it could last a lifetime. But just like the original lesion that blocked the artery, the stent may close. You must quit smoking and treat the disease process that caused the blockage in the first place. The best way to stop a stent from closing is to aggressively reduce risk factors.

Your Heart

Athletes, accomplished musicians, or experts in any field, reached their goals by learning, practicing, and working at the process. Most of them teach others and share their skills along the way. Instead of earning a promotion, a college degree or playing a musical instrument with skill, your challenge is to improve your health. By formulating a personal action plan and setting attainable goals with the help of your health practitioner, you will soon see benefits. And like other experts, you will be able to share your knowledge with family and friends.

One of the most difficult processes to change is the way you think about food. I have worked closely with many food-driven people. Many are in wheelchairs, unable to walk because of their weight. Basically trapped in their bodies, they continue to purchase and consume chips and liters of soda. It can be more difficult to change eating habits than to stop smoking. Nicotine addiction gradually wanes. We don't need nicotine to live. But food is different—we must eat. Many times a day we make choices as to what we put in our mouths.

We must not live to eat, but eat to live. Food can remain your friend but by exercising personal control, you can choose not to let food lead you down a path to ill health.

Sometimes when starting a new regimen, positive *self-talk* helps to get people through the rough parts. Tell yourself you can do it. Build your confidence.

The first step is to begin looking at food as energy instead of a reward. A prime focus in reversing heart disease is reducing inflammation. Both obesity and diabetes generate inflammatory factors that enhance arterial plaque formation. So, to reduce inflammation, improve insulin sensitivity and normalize blood glucose, weight reduction is necessary.

The primary building block in the plaque is LDL cholesterol, the lard in your arteries. Reducing the availability of LDL is mandatory. In addition, increasing HDL is just as important but is more difficult to achieve. HDL is less responsive to medical manipulation but removing saturated fats from your diet and taking a statin drug generates the ability to appropriately change both LDL and HDL to reverse disease. **Taking an effective statin, attaining normal weight and eating a low fat diet are essential. Your goal following a** heart attack is an **LDL below 70mg/dL and an HDL as high as possible.**

Many people I know look at taking a statin as a way to continue eating anything they wish, giving themselves permission to eat that bacon cheeseburger. It doesn't work that way. If you have arterial narrowing and are serious about shrinking plaques in your arteries to improve blood flow and prolong your life, you need to say good-bye to saturated fats.

Cholesterol transport is a very complex process. But simplistically, LDL delivers cholesterol into the arterial wall. HDL takes it away in a process called *reverse cholesterol transport*. HDL has the ability to mobilize cholesterol and move it out of the arteries and back to the liver. **Lowering LDL and raising HDL is not only likely to stop the narrowing, this is the reversal process.**

HDL also blocks the aggregation of platelets. Activation of platelets is the first step in forming a blood clot. Some sudden arterial occlusions occur when clots form over rough plaques inside vessels. Low dose aspirin is tolerated by most people. Its action is to inhibit platelet activity. A daily 81 milligram baby-size aspirin has been proven to decrease heart attack risk, especially if you have already had a heart attack.

HDL cholesterol particles not only act like miners removing fatty cholesterol from yellow lodes in the arterial wall, they also help block the inflammation response and increase the body's sensitivity to insulin activity. With its many valuable actions, you can see why high HDL levels are beneficial.

Daily exercise, statins, and resveratrol found in wine, grape juice, and other sources will all help to raise HDL.

The Science of Reversal

In a drug trial, Drs. Steve Nicholls and Steve Nissen of the Cleveland Clinic showed reversal of cholesterol plaques inside the coronary artery walls after 24 months of treatment. The drugs rosuvastatin or atorvastatin were used by 1,039 patients. To monitor the plaques, *intravascular ultrasonography* was used. Following the interior of coronary arteries, they were able to show reduction of plaque size. **Reversal occurred after aggressively lowering the LDL, combined with raising the HDL by at least by 7.5 mg/dL.**

Analysis of similar information by Dr. Greg Brown and co-workers at the University of Washington showed a linear risk reduction. **This means the lower the bad LDL and the higher the good HDL; the more likely you are to reverse arterial narrowing.**

Many years ago, another physician, Dean Ornish, began advocating structured lifestyle and eating transformation to a plant-based diet to reverse heart disease. People who had experienced chest discomfort because of coronary artery disease found improvement in less than a month on his recommended vegetarian diet, avoiding processed foods, combined with daily exercise. He also advocates meditation, yoga and stress reduction.

To gain the benefits of plaque reduction, it is important to set goals to limit your health risks, eat healthful foods, and normalize your lipids, blood pressure and weight. There is a transition period. As you reduce your consumption of meat products, you will miss them less. As you learn to live without fried foods and avoid buying processed foods, the changes will get easier. Soon, the smell of greasy food will be disgusting and you will easily choose alternatives.

Many people I have known who have a hundred pounds to lose were disheartened when they heard how important it was to lose weight. But, I believe the 5/2 Eating Plan may be an important one for anyone who is over weight and, through past failures, does not want to even try again. Have you heard about the 5/2 Plan? It is somewhat like deciding to quit smoking by chewing nicotine gum for two days of the week to gradually wean yourself off cigarettes.—The 5/2 Plan is not quite the same, but here's how it works.

The 5/2 Eating Plan
♥ If you look to the future in defeat and say to yourself there is no way I can lose 20, 30, 50 or 100 pounds. Ask yourself this: **Can I cut back my calories one day each week? How about cutting back two days a week?**

On the 5/2 Plan you eat about 500 calories one day, then eat a regular healthy Mediterranean cuisine or plant-based cuisine the next one or two days, then you eat only 500 calories the next day, resume regular eating the rest of

the week and repeat this ongoing. Your overall calorie intake drops gradually and you lose weight.

In 2012, Dr. Michael J. Mosley shared his concept of eating less than your usual intake for two **non-consecutive** days a week. With this plan, you reduce your calorie intake significantly but it is not as mentally challenging as setting out to sharply curtail eating for the indefinite future. His concept is to have men eat about 600 calories and women about 500 calories on two non-consecutive low calorie days.

Dr. Mosley's examples of food choices on the low-intake days are: two eggs and lean ham with water, tea or black coffee; a second meal of grilled fish or meat, with vegetables. You can make breakfast healthier by throwing out the yolks and eating a side of non-processed protein choices, such as a heap of steamed veggies. (Veggies high in protein include broccoli, mushrooms, soybean sprouts, tomatoes and onions, to name a few.)

Although fasting has been advocated for decades in many groups, harsh diets often fail miserably because metabolic changes related to starvation trigger the body to store up calories and as soon as you begin eating normally, you regain weight.

To be effective and long-lasting, the manner of eating must be sustainable. It must be a way of life — something you can do for the rest of your life. If you have a lot of weight to lose, this would be a life-changing method of gaining control of your eating and reducing weight. To review: one pound = 3500 calories. If your normal intake is 2500 calories/day and you eat 500 calories two days/week, your weight loss each week would be more than one pound. This is approximately 4-5 pounds per month and 48-60 pounds in a year. In addition, if you choose lower calorie foods, less fat and sugar, you may lose more. Most people find this plan easy to follow for long periods.

Animal studies examining the effects of fasting have shown heart benefit with reduced blood pressure and lower cholesterol levels. Intermittent fasting also lowered diabetes development in lab animals.

Because Dr. Mosley's unique concept of marked calorie reduction for two out of five days lacked scientific evidence to support the process in reduction of heart disease and diabetes in humans, I was hesitant to include it in this evidence-based book. However, as I was writing this portion of the book a very exciting scientific review in the *British Journal of Diabetes and Vascular Disease* was published!

An Aston University team in the UK, led by Dr. James E.P. Brown evaluated various approaches to intermittent fasting, looking for any evidence of advantage for its use in treating Type 2 diabetes. **In their review, they found intermittent fasting was just as effective, possibly even more effective, than daily calorie restriction and calorie counting.** Other favorable findings: markedly low calorie days (not true fasting) can reduce inflammation, reduce both glucose and lipids, and reduce blood pressure.

True fasting lowers metabolic rate and making it harder to burn fat and lose weight. Reduced metabolic rate is protective in a prolonged starvation state and impacts the ability of people today to lose weight. Researchers believe the gene pool of those who were able to survive periods of starvation has been retained in today's population. Examples are the American Indians and many Polynesian cultures that are experiencing obesity and Type 2 diabetes epidemics.

Their bodies evolved to become efficient in saving calories for harsh times. The problem today is, food is plentiful and the ability to efficiently save the energy in fat stores has become detrimental instead of life-saving.

In the 5/2 plan, eating <u>less</u> on two <u>*non*-consecutive</u> days is unlikely to lower your metabolic rate and trigger the starvation response. For example, choose Monday and Thursday as your low calorie days and add daily exercise to your weight loss plan, Exercise is an essential component to health improvement and longer life.

Pregnant women and people with Type 1 diabetes should not fast.

If you are interested in the 5/2 diet, check with your physician and obtain guidance regarding your medications during the low calorie days, especially if you are a Type 2 diabetic taking medications to lower blood glucose. Monitor blood glucose carefully and avoid readings that are too low.

There are many studies showing great benefit in delaying Type 2 diabetes, reversing glucose elevations and reducing insulin resistance with weight loss. Dr. Brown and his team are preparing clinical trials to evaluate the 5/2 dietary format as interventions in various clinical settings.

Lipid Genetic Research

Fifteen new genetic regions associated with coronary artery disease were found by an international consortium of scientists, including researchers at the Stanford University School of Medicine. At this time, scientists know there are 46 genetic links related to heart disease. Being aware of inherited links doesn't mean a magical intervention is just around the corner, but distinct progress is being made.

Within arterial plaques there is an accumulation of inflammatory cells. An unanswered question is whether the inflammatory process occurs first, triggering the accumulation of cholesterol within an artery, or occurs after the cholesterol accumulates. There are inherited mutations in key genes linked to both inflammation and heart disease. Researchers are also studying how both high blood pressure and high LDL cholesterol become key factors in the process. Updates on potential new treatments are in the news almost daily. Be sure to watch for improvements in treatment.

Medications to Lower Lipids
Statin Drugs

If so many people end up with lipid problems in adulthood, why don't we start drugs to normalize cholesterol when we are kids? Couldn't the medication simply be added to baby cereal, or bread and milk like we do vitamins?

Few treatments are that easy. Medication can be costly and produce side effects. To recommend any drug treatment, the cost/risk/benefit ratio must be considered. Is the benefit worth the money? Do the side effect risks outweigh the health benefits? Is it really worth it to expose your body to a drug that can cause harm, especially if you have no symptoms? For many people with hyperlipidemia, the answer is *yes,* because they will likely be better off taking an appropriately prescribed drug to prevent their disease progression.

Medication effects and side-effects can be safely monitored. Drugs can be changed if they are not tolerated. Pitavastatin is a new cholesterol-lowering drug that appears to be tolerated by 68% of those unable to take other statins due to side effects.

Statins are members of the primary family of drugs used to treat lipid abnormalities. Many have become generic and cost less than non-generic statins. Other than statins, additional lipid altering drugs that act on different steps in cholesterol metabolism are also available. Examples: cholesterol absorption inhibitors, fibric acid derivatives and bile acid sequestrants. At the end of this section, we will explain these options, but first, let's concentrate on the most powerful and effective lipid medications called statins.

Statins are first-line agents. They lower LDL by blocking the manufacture of cholesterol in the liver. Statins block an enzyme with a long name, shortened to *HMG-CoA reductase*. Statins are all HMG-CoA reductase inhibitors that lower total cholesterol, LDL and triglycerides while slightly increasing the good HDL cholesterol.

Many studies have documented the presence of a strong inflammatory component in the development of atherosclerosis. In some settings, a blood test, the *C — Reactive Protein* is measured to check for inflammation. One of the many beneficial effects of statins is to lower inflammation.

Some of the statin drug names are: atorvastatin (Lipitor), fluvastatin (Lescol), lovastatin (Mevacor), pravastatin (Provachol), rosuvastatin (Crestor) and simvastatin (Zocor).

Atorvastatin, lovastatin, pravastatin and simva-statin are all available in a less costly generic form. Now you know why they are called "statins" for short.

As scientists make progress in this field, more drugs will become available. For example, they are developing an antibody to be used against familial hypercholesterolemia. If successful, this disorder could be treated in those carrying the gene before cardiovascular disease occurs.

Taking measures to keep blood pressure, cholesterol, triglycerides, and weight at normal levels through proper diet and exercise is the primary approach for a longer, healthier life. When this is simply out of your grasp due to disease or hereditary factors, drugs combined with other corrective measures are recommended.

Analysis of Benefits and Risks of Statins

Although the details in this section can be tedious, we are providing this information to help you participate in your healthcare. By knowing what to ask, as well as how to answer your doctor's questions, you and your doctor can better decide the right personal course for you to take to lower your risk of heart attack and stroke. If you are not interested in the science of statin usage, skip to the end of this chapter to **Personal Support**.

As with any treatment, there are controversies and differences of opinion related to whether a person with hyperlipidemia should be treated with prescription drugs or not. In one study, 3/100 people taking a placebo (no drug) had a heart attack; while 2/100 who were on statins suffered heart attacks. So the question is: *Is it worth it to treat 100 people to prevent one heart attack?*

In 2003, a study involving nearly 20,000 people with hypertension who had at least one other risk factor, were treated with one of two hypertension treatment regimens; one with the addition of atorvastatin. **Reduction in major cardiovascular events in the group on atorvastatin was so large the data safety monitoring board terminated the study due to possible harm to those not taking a statin.**

The Lancet, a highly respected British medical journal, published a meta-analysis (evaluation of a large number of studies) where researchers examined data from 27 statin drug-trials. In a group where the LDL dropped about 40 mg/dL, they found a reduction in heart attacks and strokes. In other studies, where people who were at lower risk for vascular events, the relationship was not as clear.

Their final interpretation was: people with less than a 10% 5-year risk of having a heart attack, still benefited. A 40 mg/dL reduction in LDL cholesterol produced a reduction of 11/1000 major vascular events (heart attack or stroke). Their analysis in this group: *the benefit of taking a statin greatly out-weighed the risks.*

The Adult Treatment Panel III (ATP III) is the current evidence-based guideline arm of the National Cholesterol Education Program. Treatment guidelines are used by most physicians to guide them when treating specific lipid abnormalities as recommended by experts. This helps to standardize patient care. Cholesterol, obesity and high blood pressure recommendations are being updated and soon, an integrated guideline for cardiovascular risk reduction will be available. We need to watch for the ATP IV guide.

Using state-of-the-art information, the National Heart, Lung, and Blood Institute leads the development of guidelines for adults.

Statin Side Effects: Are your symptoms related to the drug?

Muscle pain is one of the most common reported reasons for stopping statin therapy. Muscle aching with weakness sometimes associated with statin therapy is called *statin myopathy* (*myo* - pertains to muscle; *pathy* - pertains to disease state). Those who develop muscle pain related to statins are often on high doses.

In a huge meta-analysis of 35 statin trials, there was no excess risk of statin myopathy in statins v. placebos (no drug). Yet clinical observations show muscle side effects occur and sometimes the statin must be discontinued. Rarely, severe muscle injury or kidney failure occurs. When the blood test creatine kinase is normal, there is no evidence of either progressive or permanent muscle injury. From an *UpToDate* journal analysis of numerous studies, there is about a 0.1 % occurrence of patients who experience severe myopathy. Severe myopathy is unusual with statin use.

Once you are started on statin therapy, you need to be monitored regarding its effectiveness and whether you are having any symptoms associated to its use. Even though the side effect rate is low, doctors are still concerned about undesirable effects the drug could have on your body. If you are intolerant to one drug, you may be able to take a different one.

Side effects from taking statin drugs are not as fearsome as many people believe. Other than muscle pain, reported side effects include: muscle weakness, reversible memory impairment and liver abnormalities. An additional risk is the development of diabetes. If you are taking a statin and experience muscle pain, weakness, jaundice (yellow skin) or other symptoms of concern, see your doctor right away. Sometimes reactions are due to drug interactions and not related to the statin medication alone. Blood tests are done to help assess the problem.

Many medications should not be taken with statins. Most physicians are aware of these interactions. Pharmacists also cross-check medication lists for interactions. The usual problem is interference with an enzyme that metabolizes and removes the statin from the body. If the statin is not metabolized properly, the drug level rises. The same effect results if you eat grapefruit or drink grapefruit juice — the drug is not metabolized and the blood level rises. A higher drug level may cause muscle pain.

The Food and Drug Administration recommends checking liver functions in people taking statins at two specified periods. After years of more frequent monitoring, they now recommend only a blood test soon after a drug is started, or after beginning a different drug.

Regarding memory loss from statins, you will find marked disagreement. There are reports of some older people starting on a statin followed by an abrupt onset of memory impairment. When they stopped taking the drug, memory improved. Compare this with long-term studies showing no correlation with memory loss. In fact, it is the opposite — showing taking a statin lowers the risk of dementia.

When numerous drug trials including thousands of people taking statins, were examined, a 10% increase in blood glucose was found. Based on that finding, the FDA requires a package warning to monitor blood glucose. The test, a Hemoglobin A1c, reflects the average blood glucose over the preceding three months. Blood glucose levels vary so the Hemoglobin A1c more accurately reflects the glucose level than random tests.

Justification for the Use of Statins in Primary Prevention (JUPITER STUDY)
The JUPITER study: In the *double-blind test* (where neither patient nor doctor knows if the treatment is a placebo or the active medication) the study evaluated the effect of using statin therapy to prevent cardio-vascular events and lower mortality, plus examined the risk of developing diabetes. JUPITER

findings follow, but it is important to note: statins decrease cardiovascular risk in people who have already shown health problems, such as heart attack, stroke, diabetes and hyperlipidemia when used as an additive to lifestyle change with exercise. **About the 1.7 million heart attacks and strokes occur annually in the US. Half of them happen to apparently healthy people, both men and women with low levels of cholesterol.**

Because the high incidence of apparently healthy people having heart attacks and strokes is such a huge international concern, over 1,000 doctors in 26 countries collaborated to examine this issue in association with a biomarker for inflammation. They specifically wanted to look at the benefit of taking statins for low risk individuals. Nearly 18,000 men and women with an elevated C – Reactive Protein and an LDL less than 130 mg/dL enrolled in the study.

Note: Of real importance, the (5yr) study was stopped after 1.9 years out of concern for potential harm to those receiving a placebo and no drug. Researchers in this field found the lowest cardiac event rates were seen when the LDL was below 70 mm/dL and the highly sensitive C – Reactive Protein (CRP) level was less than 2 mg/L). **There was a 54% reduction in heart attacks and a 48% reduction in strokes combined with a 20% reduction in deaths in people taking statins.** Participants followed longer than 1.9 years continued to show relative risk reduction.

Side effects in the JUPITER trial were interesting. There was no significant difference between the statin drug (rosuvastatin) and the placebo (no drug) related to muscle pain, weakness and other symptoms.

Regarding the possible development of diabetes caused by statin therapy and noted in all statins was that 80% of all the people who developed diabetes while on statins already had an elevated fasting glucose before entering the study.

Individuals with known cardiovascular disease, such as a heart attack or stroke, clearly benefit from statin therapy. It also appears people who have high lipids and high inflammatory markers would benefit from treatment even if they have no known heart or vascular disease.

157

Lowering LDL is not a full explanation for the statin benefits seen in the body. In numerous studies, there are improvements within six months. During the period when plaques were not getting smaller, researchers saw stabilization of the plaques, reduction of platelet activity related to clot formations in arteries and reduced inflammation. Actual regression of cholesterol plaques takes longer. In the Cleveland Clinic study, within two years of aggressive treatment reduction in artery narrowing was verified by ultrasound evaluations of the interior of the arteries.

Other Lipid Drugs:
There are many drugs being studied to help reduce atherosclerosis by normalizing blood lipids. As more genetic information surfaces, very specific drugs may become available in years to come. Drugs with varied activities and effectiveness are still used, sometimes in combination with a statin. However, in some cases this can cause increased side effects. Some drugs reduce lipid blood levels but are not effective in reducing heart attacks or stroke. For example, niacin was used for decades until a large study evaluating its effectiveness found there was no reduction in heart attacks or strokes; in addition there were adverse reactions. *Niacin is not considered effective.*

Other medications <u>effective</u> in modifying lipid levels in unique ways are:
- Bile acid sequestering drugs (ex. Questran/ cholestryramine) — Lowers LDL cholesterol.
- Fibric acid medications (ex. Lopid/gemfibrozil) — Lowers triglycerides and raises HDL.
- Cholesterol blockers decrease absorption from the intestine (Zetia/ezetimibe).

The reversal of cardiovascular disease requires ongoing commitment to a healthy lifestyle and proper food choices over years, over a lifetime. Atherosclerosis is a chronic disease that does not disappear. It can be controlled and with reverse cholesterol transport, HDL mobilizing LDL out of the plaques, circulation gradually improves.

Learning how to eat right, practicing healthy behaviors, avoiding excesses and exercising most days will reduce risk factors. And, if you are overweight, gradual loss of weight will help you feel better and reduce the inflammatory load on your body that enhances plaque formation.

Personal Support
Having a good relationship with your medical practitioner is very important. Monitoring many of the risk factors requires blood testing and medication management you cannot do yourself. There are many actions you can control. Sometimes, you must do what is best for you even though your family and friends are not helpful. For example: when an abstaining alcoholic is offered an alcohol drink by a "friend" — that person is not a friend. If you are diabetic or overweight and trying your best to succeed in personal changes and weight loss, yet friends and family sabotage your success by offering you foods you shouldn't eat, it makes your path steeper, more difficult. But your life depends on it. Take action. Find others interested in goals similar to yours. You can support each other.

Join a walking group Take a Mediterranean cooking class. Encourage family and friends to join you in becoming healthier. Few people are in perfect health, but to maintain health and live longer, a daily walk with a friend is a great start. If you don't have a dog but have the ability to care for one, they make wonderful walking companions. Studies also show people with pets live longer. They also have less depression and are healthier. Exercise is good for both physical and mental health. Begin by taking small steps to improve health and build on them. Change what you can change and over time, you will feel better and see your accomplishments.

You may need help from a dietician or a physical therapist. Make a personal plan to take control of your life and impact your future health by normalizing your risk factors one by one.

Primary early goals are lipid management — lowering LDL, lowering triglycerides, raising HDL; keeping blood glucose and blood pressure in normal range; daily exercise and weight reduction if you are overweight. If weight has been a problem, try the 5/2 plan. Of course stopping tobacco use is essential.

Chapter 16
YOUR HEART BEAT©

♥ **B**-Begin each morning with resolve to live healthy

♥ **E**-Eat a Mediterranean or Plant-based diet

♥ **A**-Activity – Exercise at least 30 minutes each day

♥ **T**-Teach others what you are doing-Pass it on

♥ B ♥ ACTIONS TO IMPROVE YOUR HEALTH

- Stop smoking. Stop all tobacco use. Avoid secondhand smoke.
- Maintain a normal body mass index (BMI).
- Maintain a blood pressure below 120/80.
- Keep total cholesterol below 200 mg/dL.
- Keep LDL below 100 mg/dL; below 70 mg/dL if you have heart disease.
- Maintain HDL above 40 mg/dL for men; HDL above 50 mg/dL for women.
- Consider taking 81 mg of aspirin a day/check with your doctor.
- Maintain normal blood glucose.
- Check blood work to reveal silent diseases.
- Eat only lean meat. Substitute non-fried fish for red meat.
- Avoid fried foods, trans fats and sugar.
- Seek friends with healthy habits.
- Avoid unhealthy environments.
- Avoid illicit drugs. Consume little or no alcohol.

♥ E ♥ MEDITERRANEAN CUISINE BASICS

- Eat plant-based foods: fruits and vegetables, whole grains, legumes and nuts.
- Avoid butter; use healthy oils such as olive oil and canola.
- Instead of salt, use herbs and spices for flavors.
- Limit red meat to less than once a week.
- Eat fish and poultry twice a week.

- Drink red wine in moderation (optional).

♥ A ♥ ACTION PLAN FOR FITNESS

- Be sure to consult your health practitioner before starting an exercise program.
- Begin a walking program and as your endurance increases add time and speed.
- World Health Organization recommends 3-5 hours of endurance training per week.
- If you are unable to walk — use a stationary bicycle, swim laps, do sit-ups and leg lifts, do upper-body conditioning with light weights and range-of-motion exercises.
- Consider: yoga, bicycling, consult an exercise coach or join a health club.
- Exercise daily with a friend, walk the dog, take a hike!
- Keep your mind healthy, too. Learn something new every day and remain engaged socially.

♥ T ♥ TEACH

Tell everyone what you are doing. Teach them what to do to improve their health. **Pass it on!**

Part of the process of living healthier and longer, is to establish a personal path utilizing information in *Your Heart*. If you travel this new path, take your family and friends with you. You will all feel better, find new energy and are more likely to live longer in improved health.

Change can take time — time you may think you don't have. But instead of rushing to throw a bad meal together at the last minute, you can choose to plan ahead to eat healthier. When embarking on this journey, get organized, make a list, do some shopping and consider making some meals ahead that can become your new "fast food" menu options when you are in a rush.

Take time to exercise; it lowers weight, heart risks and improves depression. Remaining physically and socially active is essential and correlates with longer life.

Betty Kuffel, MD

Chapter 17
Heart and Vessel Conditions

Your Heart is about preventing and reversing cardiovascular disease caused by arterial narrowing from cholesterol plaques. Many people have had heart attacks and live with chronic cardiovascular disorders. Some of the topics in this section address related disease processes, heart rhythm abnormalities and common treatments. A better understanding of health problems can be beneficial in recovery. This section may be used a reference point for common disorders of function, rhythm and their treatment.

Vital signs
Before covering details of congestive heart failure, let's first review the basic clinical measurements used to evaluate people. Vital signs include blood pressure, heart rate and respiratory rate. When we talk about systolic and diastolic readings of the blood pressure, the systolic (top number) is when the heart contracts pushing blood out into the aorta, while the diastolic (bottom number) is when the heart relaxes and fills readying for the next contraction.

We have already covered how to check a pulse. Normal blood pressure and pulse at rest are below 120/80 and heart rate about 70 beats per minute. Normal resting rates vary, ranging from 50-80 beats per minute. We choose 70 as a median normal rate. At rest, the respiratory rate is about 15 times per minute. Vital signs vary as an appropriate response to activity.

With increased activity such as walking or running up a flight of stairs, the heart rate increases and more blood is pumped out. The respiratory rate increases to supply more oxygen. When the heart lacks adequate coronary blood flow or the pump is inefficient, it cannot meet increased needs. If the muscle is not able to effectively pump blood out of the heart, the ability to exercise is decreased. This can trigger shortness of breath and sometimes chest discomfort.

Your Heart

Symptoms of Congestive Heart Failure

The mechanism of heart failure is complex but in simple terms, there is a reduction in ejection fraction, the forward output of blood. This causes a buildup of pressure and fluid congestion in the lungs. The ejection fraction is the amount of blood pumped out in each beat. The amount pumped out is never 100%. Normal is 55% or higher.

An ejection fraction of 50-55% is considered borderline by most cardiologists; below 50% is reduced. Imagine a heart like a saggy balloon, not pumping well because the muscle is damaged and stretched. When the contraction is weak, less blood is pushed out through the aortic valve into circulation.

The term *heart failure* scares people. Just hearing "failure" leads many people to believe their heart is going to stop altogether. It doesn't work quite that way. Congestive heart failure is usually a chronic disorder experienced over years. With advances in medical treatment, people with this problem are now living longer with less disability.

Causes of congestive heart failure are varied. Treatment is related to specific causes. We have discussed heart damage caused by a heart attack but other causative factors include: poorly controlled high blood pressure, heart valve problems and chronic ischemia with low blood flow as in coronary micro-vascular disease. The various forms of heart muscle abnormality, cardiomyopathies, also cause heart failure.

When the heart is unable to pump enough blood to supply bodily needs, fatigue is common. People with congestive heart failure can only walk short distances and often have difficulty climbing stairs. In addition to shortness of breath, leg swelling (edema) occurs. When severe, the edema can extend upward including thighs and abdomen. Sometimes it is necessary to sleep in a sitting position in order to breathe.

Congestive Heart Failure

Congestive Heart Failure is broken into: *Systolic dysfunction* and *Diastolic dysfunction:*

Systolic dysfunction occurs when the heart contracts to push blood out. In this case, the forward output, the ejection fraction (the amount of blood pumped out) is reduced. In systolic dysfunction or systolic heart failure, the left ventricle enlarges and efficiency is lost. Wall motion abnormalities are seen on an echocardiogram. Treatment includes diuretics and heart drugs. Diuretics remove excess fluid. Heart drugs help the heart contract and lower vascular pressure allowing easier ejection of blood with each contraction.

Diastolic dysfunction occurs when the heart is at rest, filling and getting ready for the next beat. This type of heart failure is not as easy to diagnose. The ejection fraction may be normal, the heart size only slightly enlarged, and yet, because the ventricle is stiff, it doesn't fill completely. Some of the causes are: high blood pressure, coronary artery disease, aortic valve disease, low thyroid and some forms of cardiomyopathy and microvascular dysfunction. Diabetes and obesity may also be factors.

We often talk about heart failure in terms of left and right. When systolic heart failure occurs and the pumping ability is impaired, fluid pressure builds and excess fluid accumulates in the lungs called *pulmonary edema*.

Heart failure can occur suddenly, such as immediately following a heart attack, but usually the condition worsens over years with lower leg swelling and increased problems breathing. In addition to breathlessness, other symptoms include: fluid weight gain, palpitations and rapid pulse. Loss of appetite may occur when venous system pressure results in congestion in the liver and intestines.

Careful management by a physician combined with patient compliance is essential. Treatment methods include: drugs to improve pumping action, a low salt diet to reduce fluid retention and diuretics to rid the body of excess fluid.

Valvular Heart Disease

From the earlier anatomy lesson, you know the heart has four heart valves that are supposed to work as one way doors. When the valves do not close properly, blood spurts through the partial valve opening. This causes turbulent blood flow and a heart murmur. When valves become diseased they may not open properly either, so the forward output of blood is limited because the opening has become too small. Blood forced through the small opening also causes a murmur. Both situations may be serious but the severity varies. Many heart murmurs are benign, requiring no treatment and are without symptoms.

Your Heart

There are many causes for valve abnormalities. As we age, our valves become stiff and some calcify. Some people are born with faulty valves. Heart attacks can result in damage to valve structures making them unable to close. Rheumatic heart disease results from an untreated *Streptococcus* infection (i.e. strep throat) and is a very serious illness that damages heart valves. *Streptococcus* bacteria can also lead to kidney damage. Today, rheumatic fever and rheumatic heart disease are not as common because access to antibiotics has improved.

Many inflammatory and infectious diseases affect heart valves. Each is treated according to cause, but sometimes surgical interventions are needed including actual replacement of valves with either mechanical or porcine (pig) valves.

During dental procedures, bacteria may enter the bloodstream. When heart valve surfaces become roughened and diseased, bacteria floating in the blood can adhere to the abnormal valve and set up an infection. Treatment is difficult, often requiring long courses of intravenous antibiotics or valve replacement.

Drug addicts who use intravenous drugs are at high risk for *endocarditis*. Look at the parts of this term for easy understanding: *endo*=inside, *card*=heart, *itis*=inflammation. When caused by bacteria it is called "bacterial endocarditis."

Cardiomyopathy

Each year about 500,000 people are diagnosed with a cardiomyopathy. This is a serious life-threatening problem involving the heart muscle. *Myo* pertains to heart and *opathy* pertains to a disease state. Some cardiomyopathies run in families. Most conditions are treatable but the complexity of diagnosing and treatment requires a skilled physician.

Heart muscle deterioration usually occurs over years due to a multitude of causes, including: viral infection in the heart muscle, nutritional deficiency, pregnancy, alcohol toxicity, chemotherapy, high blood pressure, coronary artery disease and hyperthyroidism (high thyroid hormone levels) and many inherited diseases. When no clear cause is identifiable, the disorder is called an *idiopathic cardiomyopathy*. Many cardiomyopathies are termed idiopathic. In spite of aggressive treatment, a cardiac transplant may be necessary.

Alcoholic Cardiomyopathy

Alcoholic cardiomyopathy is caused by direct alcohol toxicity to the heart muscle. It is not known why some people are susceptible to this disorder when most are not. The problem may be seen in people who do not think they drink much. Some drink only beer. The muscle becomes damaged, function decreases, heart failure occurs and the person gradually becomes disabled with fluid weight gain, shortness of breath and swollen ankles.

Palpitations, a feeling that your heart is skipping beats, or running too fast or too slow, may be the first symptom of this serious disease. The primary treatment is to stop drinking alcohol forever. Without alcohol, the heart improves, but if drinking alcohol continues or recurs, early death results.

Dilated Peripartum Cardiomyopathy

For unknown reasons, late in pregnancy some women develop dilated cardiomyopathy with systolic dysfunction called *peripartum* (near delivery) *cardiomyopathy.* When this problem occurs, the heart becomes less effective. In the weakened heart, the ejection fraction may be less than 45%, placing the mother and fetus at high risk.

Fetal distress with dire complications may occur. It is more common in twin pregnancies, also in women who develop hypertension complications with "pre-eclampsia" and in women who have had multiple children. It can occur in any pregnant woman. Some researchers believe the cause is genetic. Because fetal cells do enter maternal circulation, another theory is that these foreign cells induce a destructive inflammatory response in the maternal heart.

Some women are not diagnosed until after giving birth. Following delivery, the heart function may return to normal, but life-threatening problems may occur before the diagnosis is made. Sometimes the pregnant woman develops overt heart failure, clots inside the heart, stroke or respiratory failure. Symptoms include: palpitations, chest pain with cough, inability to breathe lying down, fatigue and abdominal pain. A cardiology consult is essential. An echocardiogram is helpful in making the diagnosis.

This life-threatening problem, identified in one US study, has a mortality rate of up to 10%. The mortality risk is higher in African American women. The causes of death are typically progressive heart failure, stroke, pulmonary embolism (blood clots in the lungs) and arrhythmias. In one study of 23 women diagnosed with peripartum cardiomyopathy, there were 3 maternal deaths and 4 heart transplants! This problem needs to be treated by highly trained specialists to provide the best possible outcome. If a woman survives and her heart function improves, another pregnancy is not recommended because of high risk for recurrence or worsening.

In addition to peripartum cardiomyopathy, viral and alcoholic cardiomyopathies, other causes include: viral hepatitis, HIV, diabetes, thyroid disease, a number of chemotherapy drugs, and the use of illicit drugs such as cocaine and methamphetamine.

Hypertrophic Cardiomyopathy

With hypertrophic cardiomyopathy the heart muscle or the ventricular septum can enlarge to the point where, when the heart contracts, the muscle-bulge is so large it obstructs the outflow of blood into the aorta, causing a sudden collapse. Loss of consciousness occurs because blood flow to the brain and heart muscle is blocked. Sudden cardiac arrest can also occur and is often the cause of death in young athletes.

Undiagnosed for years because of lack of symptoms, the problem becomes evident when the muscle reaches a critical mass, blocking outflow. A family history of sudden death in young people would suggest an evaluation of other family members. The diagnosis can be made with an echocardiogram.

Both medical and surgical treatments are available. Sometimes heart rhythm disturbances require support of a permanent pacemaker/defibrillator insertion. If a lethal rhythm occurs, the implanted defibrillator sends a shock directly to the heart muscle to normalize the rhythm.

Restrictive Cardiomyopathy

The heart becomes stiff and non-distensible; the movement is restricted. Instead of being elastic, stretchy and able to pump efficiently, the walls of the heart are infiltrated with substances. In *amyloidosis*, an abnormal protein accumulates, or in the inflammatory disease *sarcoidosis*, small masses collect in organs including the heart and lungs. This form of cardiomyopathy causes diastolic heart failure, though less common than other forms of heart muscle abnormalities, it is diagnosed with common tests.

Heart Rhythm Abnormalities and Treatment
Rhythm problems are being covered in this section because they require diagnostic procedures to make an accurate diagnosis and aid with treatment. Palpitations, feeling an irregular heart beat, may be the only symptom. Many heart problems cause irregular beats. To make the diagnosis your physician must analyze an electrocardiogram. Additional tests may be required.

Atrial Fibrillation
When the heart beat becomes irregular, most people are aware of a painless fluttery feeling in their chest. Some can sense skipped beats, both slow and rapid rhythms, but many people are unaware their heart rhythm has become irregular. If it is too fast or too slow, weakness or a faint feeling may occur. Everyone has occasional palpitations but most of the time the irregularity is benign and unrelated to atrial fibrillation.

The term *atrial fibrillation* (*atrial*=upper heart chamber, *fibrillation*=irregular rhythm) has become everyday language to many people, primarily because of treatments promoted through television ads for new blood thinners. With atrial fibrillation, there is a significant risk for stroke.

In atrial fibrillation, the upper and lower chambers no longer beat in a synchronized fashion. Instead, they beat independent of each other. Normally, the upper chamber's innate pacemaker discharges a signal stimulating an immediate contraction which empties both upper chambers into their lower ventricles. The same electrical signal in sequence next stimulates the ventricles and they contract, pumping blood to the lungs and out to the body.

In atrial fibrillation, the atria (plural form of the word) quiver and do not empty adequately. Without an organized paced beat, the ventricles contract erratically in no relationship to the atria. This ventricular chaotic rhythm may be slow or fast, symptomatic or without symptoms. It is common to feel weaker and have less endurance when in atrial fibrillation because the forward blood output by the ventricles is reduced by about 30%. This is because the atria are quivering and the blood is not flowing well and clots may form.

What causes atrial fibrillation in the normal heart?
If atrial fibrillation does occur, an underlying cause should be investigated. There may be no evidence of heart or valve disease. Common causes seen in a normal appearing heart are: overactive thyroid (*hyperthyroidism* with an elevated thyroid hormone) or underactive thyroid (*hypothyroidism* with low thyroid hormone). Both can cause atrial fibrillation. Additional causes include: excess alcohol use, *pulmonary embolism* (blood clot in the lung), and pneumonia. When these problems are treated, the atrial fibrillation typically resolves and may not recur.

Alcohol in Heart Disease and Rhythm Disturbances
Atrial fibrillation and hypertension may be caused by binge drinking. Many normal appearing hearts without evidence of coronary disease or valve problems go into abnormal heart rhythms after bouts of heavy drinking. This is so common, when atrial fibrillation occurs it is called *holiday heart or Saturday night heart.* Hearts without underlying disease are usually easier to cardiovert (shock) back to the normal rhythm but the abnormal atrial rhythm may recur.

Binge alcohol drinking is not commonly discussed, yet the Center for Disease Control and Prevention states 1 in 8 women and 1 in 5 high school girls report periodically consuming 4 to 5 alcohol drinks in a short period of time. Twice as many men binge drink, but the problem in women is often overlooked.

Sleep Apnea and Atrial Fibrillation
During sleep, people with sleep apnea repeatedly stop breathing. *Sleep apnea:* means without breath during sleep. There are two primary types: obstructive and central. *Obstructive Sleep Apnea* is most common and seen frequently in obese people where their weight contributes to the problem. However, some thin people have obstructive sleep apnea, too. In both thin and obese people the problem can be related to many factors including anatomy such as: large tongue, large

tonsils, short neck, and soft tissue relaxation in the throat. Sometimes surgical treatments are used.

The second type of sleep apnea is *Central Sleep Apnea*. In this case the breathing control center is faulty and the brain does not properly signal breathing during sleep.

In either situation, when the airway is blocked or when the brain fails to signal the person to take a breath, oxygen in the blood drops dangerously low causing cardiac irritability, reduced heart function and rhythm disturbances including atrial fibrillation. Some people who have sleep apnea have normal hearts; others have many risk factors related to obesity. Not all people who have sleep apnea snore, but many snore when the airway becomes partially blocked.

Sleep apnea is treated with an external pressure device to keep the airway open and provide supplemental oxygen if needed. The devices are *CPAP* or *BiPAP* units set up at the bedside.

The "PAP" of both terms signifies Positive Airway Pressure. (*C* is continuous, *Bi* is two). So with CPAP there is continuous pressure on air delivered to the lungs, keeping airways open. In the BiPAP device, two pressure levels are used; one pressure with inhalation, the other providing positive pressure during exhalation. The BiPAP is more often used with Central Sleep Apnea and severe obstructive apnea.

There is an adjustment phase when using these machines. You can try various masks or devices until you tolerate one and learn to live with it. Once you have become comfortable and realize how much better rested and energetic you feel wearing the device, it will become a nightly habit. If you have sleep apnea, your health depends on this device. Small portable units for travel are available.

If you believe you or someone you know has sleep apnea, evaluation and treatment are advised. Symptoms of sleep apnea include: snoring, daytime sleepiness, headaches, trouble concentrating, depression, irritability, and memory loss. Both high blood pressure and strokes may be seen. Risk for sudden death is increased in those with sleep apnea. Car accidents are more common because of falling asleep at the wheel. Sleep apnea occurs in children, too, causing reduced school performance and aggravated behavior problems. Your primary doctor can make appropriate referrals. Because heart disease and memory loss from reduced oxygen are common, the problem should be treated aggressively. Without proper treatment, the heart is stressed, rhythm changes and heart attacks are may occur.

What causes atrial fibrillation in the abnormal heart?
First, coronary artery disease disrupts normal heart function by narrowing the arteries and reducing blood flow and oxygen to the heart muscle. The damaged heart muscle becomes less able to contract. This leads to *congestive heart failure* with reduced forward output of blood. Backward pressure, congestion in the lungs, and fluid retention produce leg swelling and shortness of breath. With coronary artery disease you may also see abnormal heart rhythms because of damage to the electrical system. High blood pressure and other disorders can cause left atrial wall enlargement. Aging alone contributes to increased risk. The older you are, the more likely you are to develop atrial fibrillation.

When heart valves become calcified with age or diseased by infection, improper closure and heart failure may occur. When heart failure is present, whether it is from the above noted problems, or from myocarditis (heart muscle inflammation), the ventricles become flabby and weakened. The atria also enlarges and increases the likelihood that atrial fibrillation will occur. Atrial enlargement makes treatment more difficult than if the heart is normal.

Because coffee is a stimulant and can increase heart rate, some susceptible people may be encouraged to limit caffeine, especially if they have experienced abnormal rhythms. But, some studies of coffee drinkers show no increased risk for developing abnormal heart rhythms.

What is the prognosis for people with atrial fibrillation?
The good news is with proper treatment, people with atrial fibrillation can live as long as people whose hearts remain in a normal rhythm. If the rate is controlled by medications and a blood thinner such as warfarin is taken on a regular basis to reduce the risk of stroke, life expectancy is not decreased.

If atrial fibrillation is allowed to persist without controlling a rapid rate, ventricles weaken and the pumping action is decreased. Without a blood thinner the risk for stroke is high. Statistically, strokes are very serious, with 30-50% of people dying and another 15-30% left with permanent disability. With this potential outcome, it is very important to treat atrial fibrillation.

There are many reasons to treat this disorder:
- Rhythms that are too fast or too slow can result in loss of consciousness, weakness or a faint feeling.
- Low blood flow through the coronary arteries can reduce oxygen to the heart muscle and a heart attack can occur.
- Strokes can occur when blood clots form in the quivering left atrium, break loose and enter brain circulation.
- Instead of going to the brain, clots can enter arterial circulation and lodge anywhere.

How is Atrial Fibrillation Treated?
A procedure called an *electrocardioversion* often corrects atrial fibrillation. In this procedure, a low dose external electrical shock is applied to the chest when the patient is sedated. The shock interrupts the abnormal rhythm, allowing the body's pacemaker to fire regularly and return to a normal rate and rhythm.

Of great importance is the need for anticoagulation prior to cardioversion. Reducing clotting will decrease the risk of freeing atrial clots and causing a stroke when the beat normalizes. Electrocardioversion is not always successful. Or, it may briefly correct, but the abnormal rhythm recurs. Medications are then used to control rate and reduce risk of blood clots.

Atrial fibrillation can be treated medically in about 50% of patients. In some cases of recurrence, major heart centers use both freezing and radiofrequency (heat) to damage atrial neural circuits and stop unwanted electrical impulses. In a Mayo Clinic study in Minnesota where 245 patients with atrial fibrillation were treated with a cryoballoon (freezing method), after one year, 70% were still free of recurrence. Occasionally when other methods fail, electrical pacemakers must be implanted to support and regulate the heart rate and rhythm.

Your Heart

The actual mechanism for eliminating or reversing atrial fibrillation was not fully understood until recently. Researchers in Murray UT at the Intermountain Heart Institute developed new 3-D technology able to map electronic signals in the heart in three dimensions. With the new method, precise location of the area generating the abnormal rhythm can be identified and treated. This will make treatment of atrial fibrillation more accurate and effective, just as in other rhythm disturbances.

Large studies show aspirin is of very little value in preventing strokes in atrial fibrillation patients. More potent blood thinners must be used. The most common is Warfarin (Coumadin). There are newer effective, but much more expensive drugs offering similar benefit. Guidelines for atrial fibrillation no longer include using aspirin as a treatment.

Atrial Flutter

Similar to atrial fibrillation, in atrial flutter the upper and lower heart chambers are not contracting properly. In this disorder, the atria usually beat between 240 and 400 beats per minute. This is where the term *flutter* comes from. It describes the rapid "flutter waves" seen on electrocardiograms.

Luckily, all these beats are not transmitted to the ventricles or death would occur. With rates that high, there is not enough time for the ventricles to fill with blood, so the forward output to the body is inadequate or lost all together. The safety mechanism in atrial flutter is a variable heart block pattern where many of the electrical impulses do not reach the ventricles. For example, with a flutter rate of 300 and a conduction of 3:1, the actual pulse would be just 100 because only one beat in three is conducted to the ventricles to make the heart contract. Some patients have alternating atrial fibrillation and atrial flutter.

The symptoms, causes, complications, underlying diseases and treatments of atrial flutter are similar to atrial fibrillation. Cardioversion is used to return the rhythm to normal but the condition often recurs and must be treated with *cryo* (freezing) or heat methods to damage the run-away electrical pathways. Until the rhythm is corrected, atrial flutter patients must also be anticoagulated to prevent strokes.

Other Rhythm Abnormalities:
The normal heart rhythm is called *normal sinus rhythm, NSR.*
At rest, the normal rate is about 70 beats per minute. When the
heart loses normal rate and rhythm, the abnormalities all have
names that relate to the rate and location of the abnormality.
Cardiologists spend a lifetime sorting out and understanding
exactly what triggers the abnormal rhythms and how to stop
them. We won't spend a lot of time on this, but many people
have palpitations and become concerned. In people without
heart disease, many palpitations don't last long and occur
without any underlying disease. In general, any time
palpitations persist and are associated with symptoms such as
weakness or chest discomfort, you should seek medical care.

● **Tachycardia:** (*tachy*=fast, *cardia*=heart) A fast heart
rate may result from a high fever, running, or fear. The
increased heart rate is a normal response. In the case of chest
pain in association with tachycardia, seek medical care without
delay. Any time chest pain is a component of a rhythm
disturbance or palpitations, a heart evaluation,
electrocardiogram and other diagnostic studies are needed.

● **Bradycardia:** (*brady*=slow, *cardia*=heart) In this
situation, the heart rate is slow. The slow rate may be normal
or abnormal. Endurance athletes often have resting heart rates
below 50, sometimes in the 30s. For them, this is normal. For
all of us, when at rest or asleep, the heart rate slows. However,
people with heart disease may develop heart block and become
faint or even lose consciousness with a low heart rate. For
sustained symptomatic bradycardia, a pacemaker to maintain a
regular, faster rate may be required.

● **Supraventricular Tachycardia**: (*supra*=above,
ventricular=pertains to the lower heart pumping chambers)
Combined with *tachycardia*, these terms mean a fast heart rate
is originating in the atria, above the ventricles. The long name
and sounds scary but may not be abnormal. Physiologic
tachycardia stimulated by exercise is a normal cardiac
response. However, this rhythm may be abnormal and due to
an inherited problem in the conduction system of the heart. In
this situation, the nerves carrying the pacemaker impulses from
the atria to the ventricles are faulty, triggering rapid rhythms
not caused by a normal exercise response. Called *paroxysmal*
(periodic) *supraventricular tachycardia*, the rates are often

over 200 and result in loss of consciousness. There is high variability. Some episodes stop spontaneously or with a cough or breath-holding. Others require cardioversion or interventions to sever bypass tracts causing the fast rhythm similar to treatments in atrial flutter.

• **Multifocal Atrial Tachycardia:** (*multi*=many, *focal* derived from *foci*=sites) Instead of one pacemaker in the atrium firing off a single organized signal for the ventricles to contract, many areas in the atrium become pacemakers. Too many signals trigger a fast irregular heart beat. Instead of beating around 70 times a minute, rates are above 100. This problem is often seen in older people with chronic lung conditions and other problems causing low oxygen in the blood. Pneumonia, congestive heart failure, chronic obstructive lung disease and pulmonary embolism can lead to multifocal atrial tachycardia. Treatment is focused on improving oxygen, controlling the heart rate and treating the underlying disease.

• **Ventricular Tachycardia:** (*ventricular*=source is from the lower heart chamber) Combined with tachycardia, this fast rhythm originates in the ventricle and spreads to the rest of the heart. This is never a normal rhythm. Often seen in diseased hearts and during heart attacks, it can be a lethal rhythm requiring treatment with electrical shock. This rhythm can cause sudden loss of consciousness. If diagnosed and is recurrent, the problem is treated with an implanted defibrillator. Similar to a pacemaker, a special sensor identifies the abnormal rhythm and if rapid, delivers a shock. The shock blocks the abnormal rhythm allowing the heart to recover. Typically dual defibrillator/pacer units called *Implantable Cardioverter-Defibrillators*, ICDs for short, are surgically placed.

• **Ventricular Fibrillation:** As we noted earlier in atrial fibrillation, the fibrillation means the muscle quivers but doesn't pump. This is also the case in ventricular fibrillation. It is a lethal rhythm unless converted to normal sinus rhythm within a very few minutes. Typically seen in fatal heart attacks, it causes the person to lose consciousness. Ventricular fibrillation can be converted back to normal sinus rhythm by *Automated External Defibrillators (AEDs)*. Non-medical personnel are trained in their use and have saved many lives These devices are now on stand-by in schools, on airliners, in malls and hotels for use if someone has a heart attack and develops ventricular fibrillation.

• **Premature Ventricular Contractions:** As the name indicates, this particular beat comes from the ventricle and occurs prematurely (early). It is out of sync. When this happens, the early electrical impulse resets the body's pacemaker. This results in a slight delay giving the ventricle more time to fill than usual and that is the beat you feel. People describe feeling a "skipped" beat. Instead, what you feel is the normal beat following the abnormal early beat. In people who have known heart disease, palpitations must be evaluated fully and may require medication adjustments or other interventions. Premature ventricular contractions may be benign or dangerous.

• **Premature Atrial Contractions:** These are early beats arising in the atria. Usually benign, they can be related to stressors such as exhaustion, excess caffeine and anxiety. If recurrent, they need to be evaluated but are often fleeting or temporary and almost everyone has a premature atrial beat once in a while. In people with lung disease, premature atrial contractions are common. Treating the lung disease may improve heart function and reduce extra beats.

Recurrent palpitations in any age are cause for concern. Palpitations may be the first symptom to alert you to seek a medical evaluation is needed. An electro-cardiogram is the first step to identify the heart rhythm problem and look for abnormalities of the conduction system carrying each impulse to generate a contraction.

Heart Block

The term *heart block* does not mean the flow of blood through the heart has stopped. The term indicates the electrical circuit from the pacemaker in the atrium has "shorted" out, blocking the electrical impulse. The nerves in the heart carry electric signals to the heart muscle causing it to contract.

When the electrical activity is interrupted by a problem in the nerve fibers (the conduction system), the wave of electricity from the atrium cannot follow the nerve. So, like a stone dropped into a smooth water surface, the wave of current spreads through heart muscle like an ever-increasing circular wave. When this happens the heart still contracts but it takes longer for the electrical activity to reach its goal to make the muscle contract to pump out the blood. The slowed electrical activity can be seen on an electrocardiogram.

There are various forms of heart block. Some of them are not dangerous; others are life-threatening and require a pacemaker to sustain a heart beat within the normal range.

Pacemakers

When the rhythm of the heart is too slow or too erratic to trust, a pacemaker is warranted. Pacemakers are small electronic packs with magical capabilities designed and manufactured by micro-machinists. Micro-machinists are not tiny men like in Gulliver's Travels; they are skilled machinists who make the miniature parts that generate programmed electrical pulses to stimulate the heart to beat. The energy is supplied by a battery pack surgically inserted beneath the skin and linked to the heart by wires. The batteries last for years and are changed by surgically replacing the battery pack. Pacemaker function is checked by an external monitor. Pacemakers have saved many lives.

Vein and Lymphatic Disease

A dangerous problem encountered in veins is the development of blood clots inside the vessels. This is a high risk during pregnancy and following delivery, following abdominal and pelvic surgery, and simply from sitting for long periods. A long automobile ride or flight with prolonged sitting allows blood to pool in the pelvis and legs. This stagnation of blood encourages clotting to occur. Some inherited disorders cause intravascular clots. These disorders can be identified through specialized blood tests.

Deep Venous Thrombosis

A deep venous thrombosis is a *thrombus* (a blood clot) inside a deep vein. Sometimes this is called *thrombo-phlebitis* *(thrombo*=blood clot, *phleb*=vein, *itis*=inflam-mation).

It is important to be aware of clots in the pelvic area and deep leg veins because they are very common and very dangerous. With an improved understanding of the cause, even airlines encourage their passengers to walk or exercise in their seating areas during flights. Movements as simple as drawing circles with your feet or doing "pedal pusher" exercises by pumping your feet up and down to contract calf muscles can be beneficial to keep blood from pooling and clotting.

Another risk is having a leg fracture or sprain. Any kind of trauma to a limb can impede blood flow due to swelling and precipitate a clot. Deep venous clots can also occur in arms.

Why do we care if a clot is in a superficial vein versus a deep vein?
Clots in superficial veins tend to stay where they are and do not migrate. Deep veins have a direct route back to the heart and lungs. A blood clot in a deep vein is a serious problem.

Clot fragments may be small particles or larger pieces that resemble eels when they break off from the location where they initially form inside a deep vein. They enter the venous blood flow and are carried to the heart and lungs. The clots are filtered out in the lungs.

However, if the clot is large, it may lodge in the heart and cause sudden death. Or, it may be large enough to occlude lung vessels and block blood flow. Not only will this stop the transfer of oxygen, it can damage the lung tissue. Clots that break off from deep veins are life-threatening and immediate anticoagulation (blood thinning to stop clotting) must be started.

How do you know if you have a deep vein clot?
Initially there are no symptoms. As the clot enlarges, you may feel pressure in the area where it is forming, usually in a leg. There may be some swelling below the blockage and it will become uncomfortable to walk. If the clots develop in the deep veins of the pelvis or abdomen, you probably will have no symptoms until a clot breaks free and travels to the lungs.

Pulmonary Embolism
A blood clot in the lung is called a *pulmonary embolism*. *Pulmonary* pertains to the lung. *Embolism* is when something is floating in the blood. In this case, the clot is in a *vein* returning blood to the heart. Once through the heart it is stopped in the lung.

When a small clot lodges in the lung, if it is small enough, you may have no symptoms. If it is large or there are several of them, you will develop sudden chest pain, respiratory distress, possibly coughing and may even cough up small amounts of blood. Call 9-1-1.

Prevention is best. Because the risk of a deep vein clot is so high after orthopedic surgery including total hip and total knee replacements, it is customary to prescribe anticoagulant drugs for patients soon after surgery to prevent this serious complication from occurring. If you have unexpected swelling after a trauma or surgery, you must not wait. Consult your doctor right away.

If you have a deep venous clot that breaks loose and migrates to the lung, you may die or have serious problems. Patients with multiple traumatic injuries following an accident, or hospitalized and bedridden patients, are started on blood thinners to prevent blood clots from developing due to inactivity. Of course, sometimes, people cannot be anticoagulated because of other problems such as bleeding ulcers, head trauma or recent surgery. In most cases, anticoagulation is considered. But in trauma cases where injuries are likely to bleed and it is too dangerous to thin the blood, temporary filters resembling little umbrellas are placed inside the inferior vena cava to prevent blood clot from reaching the heart and lungs.

Once the deep clot in the vein has been diagnosed and treatment begun, the hope is to stop further clot progression and stop the risk of migration. Thinning blood is commonly accomplished with the oral drug, warfarin (Coumadin). But an injectable drug can be used for rapid effect. The minimal time for anticoagulation after a deep vein clot is three months. Depending on circumstances, it could be longer. If recurrent, or related to inherited clotting abnormalities, anticoagulation is necessary throughout life.

It is important to wear elastic support stockings to help compress the affected leg, stop tissue fluid from accumulating (edema) and improve venous blood flow back to the heart. Compression stockings help prevent *post phlebitic syndrome (post*=after, *phlebitic*=vein, *syndrome*=disorder). This is a problem in which the veins are damaged and the involved leg may swell for the rest of your life. Treatment to reduce the risk of more clots requires support hose and care to prevent further injury to the chronically swollen leg.

179

Varicose veins

Most people know what they are. Even though they look like purplish ropes under the skin in the legs, they are not usually problematic except for their appearance. These are very common and generally need no treatment. Varicose veins are unsightly and some men and women have them surgically removed. But these superficial veins are used as grafts in some coronary bypass procedures. Most doctors recommend no surgical intervention unless in cases where the veins are judged to be a risk for deep vein problems.

Lymphangitis

Although this is another new word, by now you can probably figure out this condition refers to lymph (*angi*) vessels with inflammation (*itis*). This lymph vessel condition is important to review because it is interconnected with the heart and blood vessels.

When an infection occurs within tissues, lymph fluid helps drain the area. With most minor infections, such as a small infected cut, infection-fighting white blood cells organize and assist in the healing process. However, if the infection worsens and tracks into the lymph vessels, the vessels become inflamed. Red lines leading away from the infected wound become visible on the skin. The common term for this is "blood poisoning." It is an accurate term. Red streaks indicate *lymphangitis*. Bacteria from this area enter the lymph system and are carried into large veins near the heart.

Bacteremia, bacteria in the blood, is a serious problem requiring an immediate trip to a physician for an evaluation and antibiotics. Without treatment, the problem may worsen and lead to life-threatening septic shock. In people with diseased heart valves, bacteremia can cause *bacterial endocarditis,* bacterial infection inside (*endo*) the heart. Treatment for this type of infection is difficult and usually requires weeks of intravenous antibiotics.

Lymphedema

Lymph vessel problems occur when their route back to the heart is interrupted surgically or by serious injury. The area below the injured area swells because the drainage route no longer exists. Infection in the area without lymph drainage is difficult to treat and must be protected from injury. Swelling can be significant and compression elastic garments for the leg or arm may be necessary. Women who have had breast cancer and underarm removal of lymph nodes often experience this problem and require specially fitted elastic sleeves to help control swelling.

Chapter 18
The Science of Fats

Dietary fat is a primary component of atherosclerosis and coronary heart disease. When fat consumption is high, the tendency to develop the disease early in life is increased and progresses with age. This section will provide information on types of fat, why some are more harmful than others, and which dietary choices are beneficial.

<u>Fat Structure</u>
Monounsaturated, Polyunsaturated and Trans Fat
First of all, monounsaturated fatty acids and polyunsaturated fatty acids (PUFA) are healthier than trans fats. They begin as oil, liquid at room temperature. The process of hydrogenation raises the melting point making oil become solid at room temperature, and turns oil into stick margarine. The hydrogenation process makes them unhealthy.

If oil is "partially hydrogenated," the reaction process is stopped at the point where the product is soft like some brands of margarine marketed in plastic containers. Adding hydrogen makes the oil more resistant to spoilage, prolonging shelf life.

Many commercial baked goods contain trans fats. You may already understand what trans fats are because they are frequently in the news. Trans fats are bad fats because when consumed, they raise cholesterol. Found naturally in the fat of meat and dairy products, trans fats also form during the hydrogenation of healthful plant-based oil.

(*Molecular discussion follows. Please skip the next 3 paragraphs if you are not interested in the chemistry of fats.*)

By definition, *monounsaturated fats* contain only one molecular double bond in the fatty acid chain; polyunsaturated fats have more than one double bond. Fats are called *trans* or *cis* depending on the position of the double bonds. In the hydrogenation process both cis and trans fats are formed. The trans fat configuration is a unique partially hydrogenated fat in which the molecular configuration is in the *trans position* producing a straighter molecule. This results in a higher melting point. Basically, the hydrogenation process turns healthy plant-based oils into unhealthy fats that will raise blood lipid levels when consumed.

Your Heart

Saturated fats (example: lard) are fully saturated with hydrogen; no more hydrogen can bond. However, they are not called trans fats because their bonds can rotate (not locked in the cis or trans molecular configuration). Saturated fats are solid at room temperature.

♥ Olive oil is a primary monounsaturated oil source. Olive oil contains oleic acid which has a single cis double bond. Therefore it is a *mono*–single *unsaturated fatty acid*. Olives, avocados, sunflower seeds, peanuts, almonds, whole grains, popcorn and cashews are high oleic acid. Research shows an improvement in diabetic insulin levels and blood sugar control when olive oil is used. Remember oil is caloric. Even though it is healthier than butter, one tablespoonful of any fat equals 100 calories.

Polyunsaturated fat is divided into two types: omega-3 fatty acids and omega-6 fatty acids. Primary sources of omega-6s are soy, corn and safflower oil. Omega-3s are found in canola oil, flaxseed, walnuts and cold water fish. Soybean oil contains both omega-3 and omega-6.

When you eat trans fats your LDL goes up. That results in more "lard" in your arteries. In addition, trans fats may also lower your good cholesterol. You need to keep your consumption of trans fats as low as possible. The American Heart Associations recommends limiting intake to less than 1% of your total daily calories.

Be sure to read labels. Many processed foods contain trans fats. If a serving has less than 0.5 grams of trans fat, the label may state zero. Some restaurants now advertise they are no longer using trans fats in deep frying. That is excellent news; however, any fried food contains significant amounts of oils and calories. Avoid all fried foods if you are on a calorie-restricted diet or have lipid abnormalities.

Some of the common commercial foods containing trans fats are: microwave popcorn, cake, cookies, pie, margarine, frosting and coffee creamers. If you buy commercial items, choose those containing zero trans fat. Specifically avoid partially hydrogenated oils and shortening.

Denmark was the first country to ban tans fats from foods. In 2008, California became the first state to ban restaurant chains from using trans fats for cooking; New York City and Chicago followed suit. More recently, five additional states have joined in, as have cruise ship lines and hotel chains. As a country, along with banning smoking in public places and the many Quit Smoking campaigns, we are now taking steps to change food choices to help overcome our heart disease crisis.

Cutting both trans fats and saturated fat from your diet is very important. Combine this modification with eating only lean meat and adding omega-3 fatty acids found in fish. Making these choices places you on the right track toward heart health.

♥ If you need to cook with oil, use mono-unsaturated products such as olive oil, peanut and canola oils or polyunsaturated oils. If your LDL and total cholesterol levels are high and you are overweight, avoid fatty meat, eat few egg yolks, avoid cheese and whole milk products. Consider eating veggie egg white only omelets.

Coconut Oil and Saturated Fat
Coconut oil is 91% saturated fat, 6% unsaturated and 3% polyunsaturated. Many health organizations, including the American Heart Association and the American Dietetic Association advise against eating coconut due to the saturated fat content. There is a lot of misinformation and many questions related to its consumption. Years ago the bad press was related to "partially hydrogenated" coconut oil found in powdered coffee creamers. As we know, the hydrogenation process turns healthy fats into less healthy fats.

Nutritional expert Thomas Brenna, professor of nutritional sciences at Cornell University stated non-hydrogenated virgin coconut oil may not be bad for us to consume. A large portion of the oil in coconut is lauric acid, a saturated fat that increases both HDL (good) and LDL (bad) cholesterols, but it is the ratio of good to bad that is important.

In a meta-analysis of 60 controlled trials, the conclusion was that although total HDL (good) cholesterol is a sensitive predictor of coronary artery disease risk, favorable effects of coconut fat don't exclude unknown potentially unfavorable factors. So from this huge study there are no guidelines for coconut consumption. More studies are needed.

Populations of people living in the tropics have consumed coconut as their primary source of dietary fat for centuries and had no significant heart disease or culture-wide weight problems until moving to urban environments and eating a non-native diet. Many of these populations would eat healthy fish high in omega-3 fatty acids as their primary dietary protein. The combination of their daily choices and exercise provided a healthful balance.

So, should we be eating coconut or not? Is it heart healthy? Should we drink coconut milk and avoid cow's milk and the associated animal fat? Or, is the saturated fat in coconut just as bad, or possibly even worse than cow's milk?

Researching the answers to these questions from an evidence-based standpoint was difficult. Many testimonials about health benefits are without documentation. Testimonials are meaningless.

Facts about coconut oil:

- *Lauric acid is the coconut saturated fat. It is a medium-chain fatty acid* and not a long-chain fatty acid like most fats in our diets.

- Medium-chain fatty acids (MCFAs) are different. They are absorbed and transported from the small intestine directly into the liver via the portal vein, bypassing systemic circulation.

- MCFAs are oxidized rapidly in the liver and converted into fuel burned for energy, something endurance athletes are exploring and utilizing. Increased endurance and prolonged life-span occurred in studies of animals eating medium-chain fatty acids.

- MCFAs are less likely to enter fat storage. Loss of body weight is documented in numerous animal and human studies. Improved weight loss is seen in human studies in which diets contained MCFA 24 % of calories.

- Use as cooking oil results in suppressing body fat accumulation. Coconut oil can be eaten as salad oil and used as cooking oil but if heated above 150-160 degrees, the oil breaks down.

- An animal and human study showed medium-chain fatty acid consumption resulted in a reduction of hunger and increased energy expenditure. And, when replacing long-chain fatty acids in the diet, MCFAs helped with weight control.

- The claim that MCFAs do not increase plasma cholesterol is poorly documented.

• Coconut oil is a natural antibiotic. Dental research shows it attacks the dominant oral bacteria adding to tooth decay, *Streptococci mutans*. Watch for new dental products containing coconut oil.

• Coconut milk is an antioxidant containing vitamin C and many electrolytes including potassium. Coconut water is a good sports drink (lower sodium and higher potassium) when compared with commercial sports drinks. Compare labels.

• MCFAs provide good nutritional replacements for people with malabsorption syndromes.

• Used as skin and hair moisturizer, the oil is used as a lubricant and is in soaps. Research is ongoing for additional lubricant applications, even in automobiles.

Coconuts and coconut oil both appear to be nutritious and a good choice when used in moderation. More studies examining the exact effect on blood lipids are needed. But at this time, there are many benefits to including lauric acid in your diet while also monitoring its effects on blood lipids. A 2 inch by 2 inch by ½ inch piece of fresh coconut is about 150 calories. It is crunchy, high in fiber, mildly sweet and filling.

Fat Absorption

Dietary fats take different routes from the intestine depending on their molecular structure. The short-chain or medium-chain fatty acids are absorbed directly into the blood through capillaries and are carried to the liver by the portal vein for modification. Coconut oil is about a 60% medium-chain fatty acid.

As a comparison, butter contains both short-chain and medium-chain fatty acids along with some trans-fatty acids. Some studies have suggested the short and medium chain fatty acids stimulate insulin secretion and accelerate reduction of glucose levels in the blood so may be a good oil choice for diabetics.

The small intestine has villi, fingerlike projections that absorb nutrients. In the small intestine, bile salts and pancreatic lipase act on ingested triglycerides to break them down into free fatty acids and mono-glycerides allowing them to be absorbed by the villi. Once absorbed, the fatty acids again form triglycerides and combine with carrier proteins. In the complex form, they are transported in the lymph and then into the blood where the fat molecules are carried to the liver. The liver is the processing plant, making lipoprotein forms, including LDL. This is a simple overview of a very complex process.

Essential fatty acids are fat forms not made by the body and must be supplied in the diet. Examples are *linoleic acid* and *alpha linolenic acid*; both are found in plant oils.

Read package labels. Fill up with vegetables and fruits, avoid fats. With green salads, watch salad dressing labels because many of them are loaded with fat and calories.

Review time - Normal Lipid Levels:

Total Cholesterol: 200 mg/dL or less.

LDL: 100 to129 mg/dL – If you have heart disease, the LDL goal: 70 mg/dL.

HDL: 60 mg/dL or higher – Above this level is considered best.

HDL needs improvement if HDL is below 40 mg/dL in men or below 50 mg/dL in women.

Triglyceride: 150 mg/dL or less.

Betty Kuffel, MD

Chapter 19
The Science of Sugars

Sugar consumption plays a large role in making us fat. Carbohydrates and sugars are dense with calories. If they are consumed and not needed for energy, the excess is efficiently stored in fat cells. Understanding the metabolism of carbohydrate and sugar provides a foundation for healthful food choices. A combination of eating unhealthy fats and sugars is instrumental in causing the coronary heart disease and obesity epidemics we see today. This section sorts through sugar science and sugar's contribution to weight gain and ill health.

Understanding Sugars
Sugar is a sweet chemical substance composed of oxygen, hydrogen and carbon. Pure sugar such as table sugar and cotton candy provide energy but are empty calories, and contain no vitamins or other nutrients. Fruits and vegetables contain sugar but provide nourishment as well.

Sugar is found in the "sap" of most plants including trees. Maple trees are the source of maple syrup. The high concentration of sugar both in sugarcane and sugar beets provide most of our sugar. These large cultivated crops are grown around the world and processed into sugar products.

The US Department of Agriculture reported 10,364 metric tons of sugar was consumed in the US during 2012. This translates to 136 pounds of sugar per person per year in the US. Half of this is from corn-derived sweeteners like high fructose corn syrup.

Sugar Structure
Carbohydrates are complex sugars made up of various simple sugars and are a primary source of nutrition found in products like bread and pasta. Digestion breaks down the complex molecules into simple sugars to be used as sources of energy and molecular processes in the body.

Monosaccharides (*mono*=one, *saccharide*=sugar) *Glucose, fructose and galactose* are all single molecule sugars. *Glucose* is dextrose, found in fruits such as grapes and other plants juices. Carbohydrates are converted to glucose via digestion. The sugar in blood is carried in the form of glucose and is essential for life. Glucose in the form of glycogen is stored in the liver and muscles as ready sources of energy.

The brain is a highly metabolic organ with 100 billion nerve cells called neurons. Neurons are unable to store energy, yet require glucose to function. The normal functioning pancreas of a non-diabetic person keeps blood glucose levels in a very narrow range of normal. In individuals who have diabetes, glucose regulation is faulty. Insulin is necessary to utilize sugar. However, when diabetics take insulin and do not eat, the excess insulin drops the blood glucose too low and the brain goes into crisis without a glucose energy source. At that point confusion or unconsciousness occurs. This is called an insulin reaction or *hypoglycemia. Hypo* means low; *glycemia* means blood glucose.

If the diabetic person is unable to take oral sugar because of reduced mental status (unconsciousness), intravenous glucose, or an injection of glucagon must be given to stimulate the liver to convert stored glycogen into glucose, to raise the blood level and restore brain function.

Fructose, fruit sugar, is the sweetest sugar and is one of the components of table sugar. It is also found in sugarcane, fruits, and sugar beets. Honey contains glucose, fructose and sucrose (80% sugar, 20% water).

High fructose corn syrup is frequently in the news. Using enzymes, syrup made from corn is converted into glucose and fructose. This "high fructose corn syrup" is a very sweet additive to many commercial products and beverages.

Disaccharides (*di*=two, *saccharide*=sugar); means a double sugar molecule. *Sucrose* is a sugar composed of *glucose and fructose*. Sucrose comes from both sugar beets and sugarcane. It is also found in fruits and root vegetables such as carrots. Table sugar (granulated sugar) is the *disaccharide, sucrose.*

Other disaccharides are: *maltose* and *lactose.* Both are composed of two molecular structures, *maltose* is made up of *two glucose units. Lactose,* the sugar found in milk, is composed of *galactose and glucose*. To be used by the body lactose must be broken down by the enzyme *lactase.* Many adults do not have this enzyme; they are "lactase-deficient." Unable to digest milk, they are said to be *lactose intolerant* and develop bloating and diarrhea when they consume milk products. *Galactose* is used by the body as a building block for cells. It is also an integral part of the cell structure of blood cells and is involved in A-B-O blood typing.

Maltose and lactose are found in barley where the sugar is converted to malt and in the body where sugar is digested to glucose.

Sugar Processing

Sugar beets can be processed into white sugar in one stage. Sugarcane requires multiple processing steps to become sugar.

Molasses is a byproduct of both sugarcane and sugar beet processing. It is the concentrated syrup remaining when no more sugar can economically be extracted. Rum is produced from cane molasses.

Crystals of raw sugar are brownish. Brown sugar used in baking is a step in the sugar process and can be made from sugarcane or beets, but is commonly cane-derived. Brown or raw sugar is no better than white sugar. Raw sugar is less refined and retains some brownish color from molasses in processing. The body recognizes sugar molecular structure, not the source.

High Fructose Corn Syrup

Facts: Table sugar (sucrose) is 50% glucose and 50% fructose. High fructose corn syrup is 55% fructose. The sweet syrup made from corn is used in many commercial products including protein bars and fruit drinks. Because fructose is used in many sweetened drinks, the high fructose corn syrup consumption has risen.

♥ Important facts: Fructose is part of glucose metabolism but dietary fructose is not needed. In fact, fructose is poorly absorbed and not used as an energy source in the same way as glucose. The liver, instead, processes fructose in a method favoring *lipogenesis* (fat production). Studies in animals and monkeys show when they eat diets high in fructose and sucrose, they develop hyperlipidemia. The American Journal of Clinical Nutrition published a Swiss research article showing overweight school children had higher blood lipids, lower HDLs and their LDL particle sizes were small. More studies are needed to identify the exact reasons why high fructose consumption correlates with obesity and cardiovascular risks.

There is no nutritional reason to consume fructose and it appears to be harmful.

High fructose corn syrup is higher in fructose because the processing removes part of the glucose in the mix by converting it to the sweeter fructose. Table sugar from any source contains 50:50 (glucose and fructose). **However, in the body there is a big difference between glucose and high fructose corn syrup in the way it is metabolized.**

Italicized for emphasis:

• *When the brain utilizes glucose, MRI scans document increased activity in a part of the brain called the hypothalamus. Brain activity is followed by a rise in ghrelin and other neuropeptides known to **suppress appetite**.*

• *When fructose is consumed, you remain hungry because there is no rise in appetite-suppressing substances. Fructose is metabolized via a different pathway in a process that also generates uric acid and can stimulate gout. Without the release of ghrelin, you remain unsatisfied in spite of consuming significant calories.*

• ***Diabetes, obesity and metabolic syndrome correlate with consuming fructose.***

Many studies have examined the impact of sugar on the brain, the body and the pancreas. Studies are on-going and we will hear more evidence in the future. The bottom line is: avoid sugared drinks. They are high calorie and do not contribute to health. One cup of fresh orange juice contains 112 calories and 20 grams of sugar. The natural sugar in OJ is sucrose (one molecule of fructose and one of glucose).

Many soft drinks have lower sugar content than juices. Be sure to read labels. If a juice is not 100% juice, by regulation of the FDA it is labeled as a *juice drink or juice cocktail*. The label may say "no added sugar" yet the drink could contain a large amount of natural sugar. You are much better off drinking a glass of water and eating a nutritious 70 calorie orange with its fiber than drinking bottled juice of any source.

Does sugar make kids hyper?

Three large studies say — *No.* In a large analysis of the association of sugar and hyperactivity in children published in the Journal of the American Medical Association including sixteen studies, this meta-analysis of all these studies found NO sugar effect on behavior or cognitive performance in children.

In an article in the British Medical Journal, examining a dozen double blind studies, there was no detectable difference in children getting sugar or not. Sugars included: chocolate, sweets and natural fruit sources. These studies included some children with hyperactive attention deficit disorder.

Substances in soft drinks such as the stimulant caffeine could add to some behavior changes. Study subjects evaluated had consumed known quantities of sugar, compared with placebo (no sugar) and the studies were "blinded" so the children, the parents, the observers and research staff did not know who was given sugar-containing substances.

Studies on sugar consumption in children reported in the New England Journal showed no behavioral changes in children consuming cake, sweets, candy and sugared drinks. The conclusion was — there is no such thing as a "sugar high." If a food or drink contains a large amount of caffeine, there is reason for being more alert or stimulated. Following food intake, blood glucose rises a few points but with proper insulin function (non-diabetic) within two hours the elevation has resolved.

Is sugar okay for kids?

Even though there is no validity to the concern that kids get high or hyperactive on sugar, fresh fruit options should be substituted for sugary desserts, candy and sweet drinks. High sugar consumption contributes to obesity and poor eating habits. Occasional sweets are fine for non-diabetics, but regular exercise and teaching the importance of eating healthful foods are goals beginning in childhood. Remember, pure sugar such as table sugar and cotton candy provide energy but are empty calories and contain no vitamins or other nutrients. Fruits and vegetables contain sugar but provide nourishment as well.

Your Heart

SUMMARY

Coronary artery disease and the development of atherosclerosis throughout the body begin in childhood. Now is the time to teach children healthy food choices and to lead active lives. By learning this information, you can begin by making sound choices for yourself, but don't stop there, spread the information to family and friends. Don't forget your pets; they develop the same diseases as their overweight human caretakers. Food, exercise and health choices you make today can help prevent cardiovascular disease, obesity, diabetes and other related diseases in the future.

Your Heart is full of up-to-date evidence-based health information — researched and reviewed right up to the date of publication. As more studies are released and as health recommendations change, the YourHeartBook.com website and blog will provide frequent heart health updates.

Lifestyle practices, exercise options to improve cardiovascular health and healthful food choices are actions you can take *right now.* By following the Lipstick Logic Cardio-Action Plan and Your Heart BEAT© options, you will feel better, your heart will be healthier, and you may add years to your life.

Betty Kuffel, MD

Acrolein-an active harmful substance in cigarette smoke contributing to atherosclerosis

Alveoli-tiny air pockets in lung tissue where oxygen-carbon dioxide exchange occurs

Anabolic Steroid-a hormone related to male characteristics

Andropause-male aging with reduction in testosterone production

Aneurism-weakness in an artery resulting in thinning, bulging and possible rupture

Angina-chest pain resulting from lack of oxygen to the heart muscle

Antioxidant-a substance that supplies electrons to neutralize free radicals, reducing cell injury

Aorta-the largest artery

Arteries-blood vessels with muscular walls carrying oxygenated blood throughout the body

Arterioles-tiny arteries that join capillaries

Atherosclerosis-accumulation of cholesterol within artery walls causing narrowing

Atrial fibrillation-abnormal irregular heart rhythm with atria and ventricles lacking synchrony

Atrial flutter-abnormal heart rhythm with rapid irregular beats

Body Mass Index (BMI)-mathematical formula used to estimate body fat

Bradycardia-slow heart rate

Brain attack-brain stroke

Capillaries-tiny blood vessels where transfer of nutrients, wastes and oxygen exchange occurs

Cardiomyopathy-heart muscle abnormality

Cardiopulmonary bypass-machine supports circulation and oxygenation during heart surgery

Cardiovascular Disease-cholesterol accumulates within the inner artery wall

Celiac disease-autoimmune destructive process in the small intestine due to gluten intolerance

Cerebrovascular Accident-stroke

Cholecalciferol-a form of vitamin D

Cholesterol remnant particles-harmful lipid associated with high triglyceride

Your Heart

Cholesterol-fat/lipid measured in blood, found in animal fats, contributes to atherosclerosis

Cocaine-illicit harmful stimulant drug resulting in significant arterial damage

Collateral circulation-arteries near areas of blockage enlarge and improve blood flow

Congestive heart failure-pump action of heart is impaired often causing lung congestion

Coronary microvascular disease-atherosclerosis of small arteries in the heart muscle

Coronary sinus-large heart surface vein carrying blood from heart muscle to atrium

C-reactive protein-a blood test for inflammation

Deep Venous Thrombosis-a blood clot in a deep vein; thrombosis=blood clot

Defibrillator-machine that delivers a precise electrical shock to treat abnormal heart rhythms

Diastolic-lower number of blood pressure; relaxation phase of heart beat

Echocardiogram-ultrasound examination of the heart, vessels and valves

Ejection fraction-volume of blood pumped out with each heart beat; normal is 55% or higher

Electrocardioversion-treatment of abnormal heart rhythm using low dose electrical shock

Endocarditis-inflammation/infection inside the heart

Essential hypertension-the most common kind of high blood pressure

Estrogen-female hormone

Exertional angina-heart pain from reduced oxygen/blood flow with activity; resolves with rest

Free-radicals-unstable molecular substances that damage cells, reduced by antioxidants

Gliadin and Glutenin-products in wheat grains, especially gliadin, causing celiac disease

Gluten Intolerance-body has developed inability to consume and tolerate wheat products

Gluten-sensitive or gluten-reactive-when people test negative for celiac disease but become ill from eating wheat products

Heart block-electrical abnormality when nerve conduction of heart beat is impaired

Heart failure-heart muscle pumping action is impaired; fluid accumulates in lungs

Hemorrhagic stroke-brain hemorrhage from ruptured artery causing a stroke

High Density Lipoprotein-HDL-cholesterol is the "good" cholesterol, high is good

Hypertension-high blood pressure

Hypertriglyceridemia-elevation of one of the blood fats-triglycerides

Hysterectomy-surgical removal of uterus

Insulin resistance-when muscle, liver and other cells don't respond to normal levels of insulin *Insulin*-hormone produced by the pancreas essential for the utilization of glucose

Lipids-blood fats, cholesterol and triglycerides

Lipoproteins-the way fats are transported in the blood bound to proteins

Low Density Lipoprotein-LDL-cholesterol, the "bad" cholesterol; you want it low

Lymphatics-thin vessels carrying lymph fluid

Macrophages-a white blood cell form involved in immune processes and atherosclerosis *Marijuana*-currently illicit except for medical use; psychologically addictive drug

MDPV (methylenedioxypyrovalerone)-illicit dangerous stimulant drug, common name *bath salts*

Mediterranean Diet-healthful diet consumed by people bordering the Mediterranean Sea

Metabolic syndrome-body process seen with obesity, insulin resistance and high cholesterol

Methamphetamine-illicit highly addictive destructive stimulant drug

Multifocal Atrial Tachycardia-chaotic rapid heart rhythm

Multi-infarct dementia-memory impairment resulting from multiple small strokes

Myocardial infarction-heart injury due to lack of oxygen/blood flow=heart attack

Osteopenia-reduced bone density

Osteoporosis-advanced state of reduced bone mineral, weakening, fracture risks

Your Heart

Paleo diet-Paleolithic diet; "caveman" diet of fresh produce and range-fed meat

Plant-based-the new name for vegetarian eating

Premature Atrial Contractions-early irregular heart beats originating in atrium, usually benign

Premature Ventricular Contractions-early irregular heart beats, originating in ventricle, may be benign or pathologic

Progesterone-a hormone produced by ovaries

Pulmonary edema-fluid in the lung tissue

Pulmonary embolus-blood clot carried in the blood to the lung, dangerous, sometimes deadly

Secondhand smoke- smoke inhaled by a nonsmoker from contaminated environment

Sleep apnea-breathing cessation during sleep; obstructive airway or lack of brain signal

Smokeless tobacco-non-smoked tobacco absorbed through oral mucus membrane

Statins-shortened name for many medications used to reduce lipid/cholesterol abnormalities

Stress echocardiogram-ultrasound image of the heart performed immediately following a treadmill stress test

Supraventricular Tachycardia-rapid heart rhythm originating above the ventricle

Surgical menopause-the ovaries are surgically removed, hormone production stops abruptly

Systolic-upper reading of a blood pressure, the result of heart contraction pushing blood out

Tachycardia-rapid heart rate (fast pulse)

Takotsubo Cardiomyopathy- Broken Heart Syndrome-heart muscle abnormality seen in postmenopausal women who experience extreme stress such as the loss of a loved one

Testosterone-male hormone

Thrombolytic therapy-clot melting drug used sometimes in heart attacks and strokes

T-Lymphocytes-circulating white blood cells involved in atherosclerosis

Transient ischemic attack (TIA)-a temporary loss of neurologic function, stroke-like; resolves

Triglyceride- a fat or lipid, 2 forms: Circulating and Adipose (fat stored in tissue)

Troponin-a measurable protein released into blood by dying
    heart cells following a heart attack

Vascular dementia-memory impairment from lack of oxygen
    due to disease in brain arteries

Vasodilation-smooth muscle relaxation in blood vessels
    allowing more blood flow; lowers BP

Vegan-plant-based diet excluding all animal-derived foods

Veins-blood vessels carrying oxygen depleted blood and cell
    waste products back to heart

Ventricular fibrillation-quivering, non-beating heart, fatal
    rhythm unless shocked/defibrillated

Ventricular tachycardia-rapid heart rhythm originating in
    ventricle; often seen in heart attacks

Venules-tiny veins connected to capillaries, receive blood from
    tissues

Visceral fat-metabolically active fat accumulated around
    internal organs, increase heart disease

Xanthelasma-flat yellow plaques in skin around eyes,
    correlates with heart disease

Your Heart

REFERENCES

Risk Factors

American Diabetic Association Clinical Practice Recommendations 2013.

American Journal of Clinical Nutrition (January 2013 online) French study showing correlation of Type 2 diabetes and diet soda.

American Journal of Nutrition, Deborah Sellmeyer, MD; Animal protein consumption and bone loss.

Annals of Internal Medicine (May 2013) Published US Preventive Services Task Force recommendation for vitamin D and calcium supplements.

British Medical Journal (February 27, 2013) First signs of heart disease seen in newborns of overweight/obese mums. ScienceDaily.com

Cochrane systematic review, meta-analysis of randomized trials published in *BMJ*, 2013. Re: salt and potassium intake.

Columbia University Medical Center (2012, December 21). New insights into how immune system fights atherosclerosis. *Science Daily*.

Cell Press (April 4, 2013) Obesity without the health problems? There could be a way. *Science Daily.*

Diabetologia 2013, Author Dora Romaguera, PhD and colleagues at the Imperial College London, UK; Type 2 diabetes risk related to soda consumption.

International Agency for Research on Cancer, World Health Organization - *IARC Handbooks of Cancer Prevention*, Vol. 11, 2007, p 11: Tobacco Control: Reversal of Risk after Quitting Smoking.

Journal of the American Medical Association 2011; 305:2448-55, Authors Grontved, A and Hu, FB, Meta-analysis– Television viewing and risk of Type 2 diabetes, cardiovascular disease and all cause mortality.

Journal of the American Medical Association 2012; 308(23): 2489-2496, Gregg, EW, et al: Association of an intensive lifestyle intervention with remission of type 2 diabetes.

Journal of the American Medical Association Network Online in JAMA Internal Medicine, (February 2013) Calcium intake study.

Betty Kuffel, MD

Public Library of Science 2013, Author Sanjay Basu et al: Sugar availability and Type 2 diabetes.

NIH-MedlinePlus, American Heart Assn. spokesman statement re: calcium.

Women and Heart Disease:

Centers for Disease Control and Prevention.
www.cdc.gov/reproductivehealth

Circulation: Arrhythmia and Electrophysiology 2012; 5: 1091-1097 Smoking, Smoking Cessation, and Risk of Sudden Cardiac Death in Women.

BJOG: An International Journal of Obstetrics and Gynecology.
www.bjog.org

British Medical Journal 2012; 345 (Oct 09 2): e6409, L. L. Schierbeck, et al, Effect of hormone replacement therapy on cardiovascular events in recently postmenopausal women: randomized trial.

British Medical Journal (February 2013) Dr. Karl Michaelsson, et al, Uppsala University in Sweden Re: increased cardiovascular deaths in women on calcium supplements.

British Medical Journal (March 2013) No clear evidence that decline in hormone replacement therapy use linked to fall in breast cancer.

Tokai Journal of Exp. Clinical Medicine (Sept 2009); 34(3):92-8 Department of Obstetrics and Gynecology of Specialized Clinical Science at Tokai University School of Medicine in Japan, Hormone replacement impact on bone health and cholesterol levels.

Public Library of Science ONE, 2013; 8 (1): Ambrosi, CM, et al, Washington University in St. Louis Genes provide clues to gender disparity in human hearts.

Men and Heart Disease:

British Medical Journal Open (2013) Japanese meta-analysis on hair loss as a heart disease marker.

European Society of Cardiology (ESC) (May 2013). Heart failure accelerates male 'menopause'. *Science Daily.*

Journal of the American Medical Association (1971) 216:1185, McNamara et al: Coronary Disease cohort study on

American soldiers in Korean War – 77% with disease extending into young age groups by the mid-1950's.

Journal of the American Medical Association (May 1971) 216: 1185-877, McNamara et al: Vietnam casualty postmortems showed 45% with atherosclerosis.

Journal of the American Medical Association 1953; 152 (12): 1090-1093: Coronary disease among US soldiers killed in action in Korea.

Journal of the American College of Cardiology (Aug 1993); 22(2):459-67 Joseph, A et al, Manifestations of coronary atherosclerosis in young trauma victims, autopsy studies.

Atherosclerosis (Apr 2001); 155(2):499-508, Schmermund, A et al: Coronary atherosclerosis in unheralded sudden coronary death under age 50: Histopathologic comparison with 'healthy' subjects dying out of hospital.

Minneapolis Heart Institute Foundation report 2013.

Children and Heart Disease:
University of Eastern Finland (April 2013). Metabolic disorders predict the hardening of the arterial walls already in childhood. *Science Daily.*

Bogalusa Heart Study 1972-2005 – Cardiovascular Risk factor research, multidisciplinary team, studied hereditary and environmental aspects of early coronary artery disease for more than 30 years.

Tulane.edu/som/cardiohealth/materials.cfm

Interventions:
American College of Cardiology's 62nd Annual Scientific Session, report from Charles University in Prague, Czech Republic: Examination of off-pump by-pass in high risk patients.

National Institutes of Health abstract by V.R. Challa, MD, Dr. Challa; Cognitive decline after cardio-pulmonary bypass procedure.

Exercise:
American College of Sports Medicine (May/June 2013), 77, 3:8-13, Klika, B, Jordan, C : High-Intensity Circuit Training Using Body Weight: Maximum Results With Minimal Investment.

Betty Kuffel, MD

The Journal of Physiology (February 2013), 591, 641-656.
Cocks, Matthew, Wagenmakers, A, et al Liverpool John
Moores; University, Sprint interval and endurance
training.

Food:
American Journal of Nutrition (May 2003), 77:1146-1155,
Mensink, RP et al: Effect of dietary fats on HDL
cholesterol and serum lipoproteins.
American Journal of Clinical Nutrition (2007), 86:1174–8;
Bray, G: How Bad is Fructose?
*American Journal of Clinical Nutr*ition (November 1996), Vol.
64 No. 5 De Oliveira e Silva, ER, et al: Effects of shrimp
consumption on plasma lipoproteins.
American Journal of Medicine (October 2012), High
antioxidant diets result in lowest risk for heart disease.
British Journal of Diabetes and Vascular Disease (April 2013)
Brown, James E., Michael Mosley and Sarah Aldred,
Intermittent fasting: a dietary intervention for prevention
of diabetes and cardiovascular disease?
British Medical Journal (May 2012) Dark chocolate benefits in
heart disease.
Endocrine Society (May 2013) Fish oil supplements may help
fight against type 2 diabetes.
JAMA 2004;292:1433-1439, Knoops, KT et al, The HALE
project, Mediterranean diet, lifestyle factors, and 10-year
mortality in elderly European men and women, 50%
reduction in all cause mortality.
Journal of Nutrition (Mar 2001): 132(3):329-32 from the
School of Dietetics and Human Nutrition, McGill
University. Medium-chain fatty acids help weight control.
Mayo Clinic Proceedings online (2013), Di Nicolantonio,
James, J: L-Carnitine in the Secondary Prevention of
Cardiovascular Disease: Systematic Review and Meta-
analysis.
Nature Medicine 2013; Digestive bacteria of meat-eaters
change carnitine to product that promotes atherosclerosis.
New England Journal of Medicine 2013; 368: 1800-1808 –
Fish oil and heart risk factors.
Penn State (May 2013. Whole walnuts and their extracted oil
improve cardiovascular disease risk. *Science Daily.*

Your Heart

The Fast Diet, 5:2 Intermittent marked calorie reduction on 2 non-consecutive days per week. Mosley, Michael: The science behind the 5:2 diet. www.thefastdiet.co.uk

World Health Organization's *Codex Alimentarius* guidelines on food.

Reversal of Heart Disease:
Circulation 2007; 115: 1824-1826, B. Greg Brown, MD, PhD: Editorial-Atherosclerosis measurement.

Journal of the American College of Cardiology (Aug 2004) 44(3):720-32.: Evidence-based cholesterol guide-lines.

Lancet, (November 2010); 376(9753): 1670–1681. Statin use is highly beneficial.

New England Journal of Medicine (December 2011); 365:2078-2087, Nicholls, Stephen J., Nissen, Steven E., et all, Cleveland Clinic: Effect of Two Intensive Statin Regimens on Progression of Coronary Disease.

New England Journal of Medicine 2008; 359:2195-2207, Ridker, Paul M et al, Landmark JUPITER Study showing prevention of cardiovascular events with use of statin therapy.

Betty Kuffel, MD

ACKNOWLEDGMENTS

Your Heart is dedicated to my parents, Gordon and Lila Church. My father, even while suffering with heart disease, provided love, support and encouragement to *get a good education* but didn't live long enough to see me graduate from nursing, and later from medical school. My mother worked hard all her life, served nutritious meals, ate well, never smoked and lived to be 89. She was an advocate for women and set a positive example of love and strength for all who knew her.

With sincere appreciation, I want to thank my medical, nursing and writing colleagues who read *Your Heart* prior to publication. Their generous contributions of time and professional suggestions were very helpful. In special recognition, I want to thank Deb Burke, Lavonne Mueller, Barb Palmer, Larry McHugh, Maura Fields, RN, Cheri Zao, MD and Suzanne Daniell, MD, for their feedback and belief in this book.

My sincere gratitude also goes to other family members and friends who read, provided suggestions for clarity, and sincere encouragement to publish *Your Heart,* and I'm especially indebted to my husband, Tom, for his support and technical publishing assistance.

Finally, I wish to pay tribute to the energy, skill and devotion of my manuscript editor and sister, Beverly Erickson of Blue Heron Loft, who formulated the idea for this book and encouraged me to write it. Bev created the artwork and cover for *Your Heart.*

Your Heart

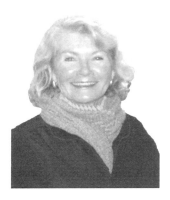

Bev Erickson

Bev has spent 25 years in marketing and public relations working with businesses ranging in size from small non-profits to large financial conglomerates. She serves as a director of two arts boards, is a member of two writers groups, Toastmasters International and the League of Women Voters. Bev enjoys writing, editing, photography, multi-media art, creating book cover designs at BlueHeronLoft.com, world travel with her husband and entertaining family and friends at the cabin she and her husband built.

Bev's education includes communication graduate studies at the University of St. Thomas, graduate of the University of Minnesota, School of Journalism, graduate of the Institute of Children's Literature and nursing graduate of Golden Valley Hospital School of Nursing.

Betty Kuffel, MD

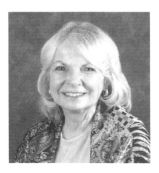

Betty Kuffel, MD FACP
An honors graduate of the University of Washington School of Medicine, Internal Medicine physician and former nurse practitioner, Dr. Kuffel has broad healthcare experience. After years of directing and working in emergency departments, she changed her focus to found and direct hospitalist inpatient care at North Valley Hospital. Recently Dr. Kuffel retired to pursue many interests including writing this educational health series for women.

Because of a shared desire to help women of all ages achieve healthy fulfilled lives, she joined with her sister Bev and founded Lipstick Logic ™ to bring health and lifestyle education to women. Their contributions to educating women include hosting and speaking at women's conferences, writing a health blog on LipstickLogic.com and writing a monthly health column for Montana Woman Magazine.

Dr. Kuffel's success in her lifetime commitment to helping others achieve optimum health has been recognized. In 2010, she was named the first Champion physician at North Valley Hospital in Whitefish, MT. In 2013, the local chapter of the Soroptimist International women's organization honored Dr. Kuffel with the Ruby Award for her professional and personal efforts making extraordinary differences in the lives of women and girls.

The Lipstick Logic concept evolved over years of caring for women in crisis. Dr. Kuffel believes education is the key to living healthier and making informed choices. Heart disease is the focus of the Lipstick Logic Volume One guide to better health because coronary artery disease is the number one cause of death and it is preventable.

206

UPCOMING LIPSTICK LOGIC HEALTH SERIES

Lipstick Logic Volume II
Your Weight: Obesity, Metabolic Syndrome and Weight Control
Within this text, obesity in both adults and children is the focus.

Obesity is a major problem threatening health in more than a third of the adult population. This volume covers the impact of weight gain on body functions and the related development of Type 2 diabetes, previously a disease of older adults. Now, nearly 20% of children are obese and, like adults, over-weight kids are developing diabetes, high blood pressure and heart disease.

This important topic was chosen for the second book because of the urgent need to modify the eating habits of America. Heart disease, stroke, Type 2 diabetes and some cancers increase with obesity. Many of these diseases are preventable or can be delayed by learning what to do and taking action to change lifestyle and eating habits. Volume II will provide you with tools and science-based relevant information as a foundation for making healthier choices.

Additional topics under consideration: Brain, Breast, Contraception, Fear, Hepatitis, Longevity.

NUTRIENT SOURCES QUICK REFERENCE
MAKE A COPY FOR YOUR REFRIGERATOR DOOR

♥ **Calcium:** Broccoli, green leafy vegetables, tofu, fortified soy milk, soy beans, baked beans, fortified orange juice, cheese, milk, nut milks and coconut milk, enriched grains and breads, fortified cereals (ex. Total, Raisin Bran, Corn Flakes).

♥ **D-Vitamin:** Found in supplements, sunshine and foods. Foods: Many are fortified with vitamin D. Read labels. Fortified foods: cereal, milk, orange juice, yogurt, margarine. Some natural sources: ocean fish, cod liver oil, egg yolk, beef.

♥ **Fiber:** Foods high in fiber tend to be filling and satisfy the appetite longer. Vegetables: cabbage, carrots, celery, chickpeas or Garbanzo beans, spinach, mushrooms, peppers, avocados, sweet corn, artichoke, broccoli, celery, eggplant and lettuce. High fiber fruits: bananas, berries, kiwi, oranges, pears, prunes. Don't forget nuts.

♥ **Fruits:** Apple, apricot, blueberries, cantaloupe, cherries, coconut meat, coconut milk, grapes, honeydew melon, kiwi, lemon, orange, peach, pineapple, raspberries, tangerine watermelon (These are lower in natural sugar and calories than many others.)

♥ **Grains (High in fiber, antioxidants, vitamins, magnesium, iron)** Oatmeal, corn, whole wheat, brown rice, barley, sorghum, millet, spelt, rye and quinoa are all great choices; also popcorn is a good choice if you omit salt and butter.

♥ **Magnesium:** Spinach, nuts, oatmeal, beans, halibut

♥ **Phosphorus:** Fish, nuts, and cereals

♥ **Potassium:** Potatoes, oranges, orange juice, melons, spinach, mushrooms, dried apricots, yogurt, salmon, avocados, bananas, beans, raisins and molasses

♥ **Protein:** Vegetables: asparagus, cauliflower, broccoli, Brussels sprouts and corn. Beans and legumes provide primary protein used as a meat substitute in vegetarian diets. Chick peas, nuts, pumpkin, squash, mushrooms; tofu and tempeh (soy foods); quinoa and sunflower seeds are all good choices. Animal sources: Meat, fish, eggs.

ENVIRONMENTAL WORKING GROUP'S ORGANIC FOOD RECOMMENDATIONS: BUY ORGANIC WHEN POSSIBLE: kale, lettuce apples, celery, sweet bell peppers, peaches, strawberries, blueberries, imported nectarines, domestic cucumbers, spinach, green beans, potatoes, grapes

CLEAN-LOWEST IN PESTICIDES: onions, sweet corn, pineapples, avocado, cabbage, sweet peas. asparagus, mangoes, eggplant, kiwi, domestic cantaloupe, watermelon, grapefruit, mushrooms, sweet potatoes